# PSYCHOLOGY AND HUMAN REPRODUCTION

# CONTRIBUTORS

*Lawrence G. Calhoun, Ph.D.*

Clinical psychologist and Associate Professor of Psychology at the University of North Carolina at Charlotte.

*Mary Lynne Calhoun, Ph.D.*

Director of Interdisciplinary Training at the Human Development Center at Winthrop College.

*Edith Saparago Irons, Ed.D.*

In private practice in Charlotte, North Carolina.

*Joanne M. Jones*

Student in the Department of Psychology, University of North Carolina at Charlotte.

*H. Elizabeth King, Ph.D.*

Clinical psychologist and Associate Professor of Psychiatry at Emory University School of Medicine, Atlanta, Georgia.

*James W. Selby, Ph.D.*

Clinical psychologist and Associate Professor of Psychology at the University of North Carolina at Charlotte.

*Ignatius J. Toner, Ph.D.*

Associate Professor of Psychology at the University of North Carolina at Charlotte.

*Albert V. Vogel, M. D.*

Assistant Professor of Psychiatry at the University of New Mexico Medical School.

# PSYCHOLOGY AND HUMAN REPRODUCTION

James W. Selby, Lawrence G. Calhoun, Albert V. Vogel, and H. Elizabeth King

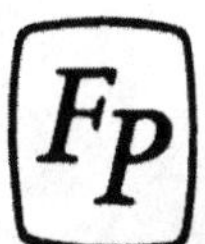

**THE FREE PRESS**
*A Division of Macmillan Publishing Co., Inc.*
NEW YORK
Collier Macmillan Publishers
LONDON

The Free Press
A Division of Macmillan Publishing Co., Inc.
866 Third Avenue, New York, N. Y. 10022

Collier Macmillan Canada, Ltd.

Library of Congress Catalog Card Number: 80-1641

Printed in the United States of America

printing number

1 2 3 4 5 6 7 8 9 10

ISBN: 1-4165-7771-8 ISBN: 978-1-4165-7771-3

James W. Selby: *To Susan, Sara, and Jacob Selby*

Lawrence G. Calhoun: *To Roberto Coimbra, Antônio Quinan, Alvin Smith, and Abraham Tesser—outstanding teachers and good friends*

Albert V. Vogel: *To my father, Victor Hugh Vogel*

H. Elizabeth King: *To Abraham Tesser, Jacob Christ, and Sarah Brogden*

# Contents

# Preface

PROFESSIONAL INTEREST IN HUMAN SEXUALITY has burgeoned in recent years, with numerous books and journals being devoted to the subject. Much of this work has focused on levels of sexual satisfaction, patterns of sexual gratification, sexual identity, and associated role behavior. Within this rapidly expanding literature, a dimension receiving far less concerted attention has been reproduction.

Events fundamental to the reproductive life cycle (e.g., pregnancy, labor, and delivery) have been the target of medical advances and yet have attracted relatively little systematic attention from behavioral scientists. Psychological, psychiatric, and social aspects of such events have often been overlooked or minimized. The research and theory that have emerged tend to focus on a particular event, such as pregnancy, without a context of the reproductive cycle as a whole. Consequently, there has been minimal integration into an overall framework. Within the present volume, psychosocial aspects of a number of major events within human reproduction are discussed.

The introduction provides a conceptual structure and orientation. Major reproductive events are presented as issues in living encountered by most people. These events are viewed as potential hazards for personal and social adjustment, which some people negotiate with relative ease; others experience mild, moderate, or severe distress when confronting them. Subsequent chapters each focus on a particular event such as pregnancy, delivery, or the postpartum period and examine the available data and professional thinking concerning the psychological and social dimensions of that event. In every chapter an attempt is made to provide a review and a critical analysis of empirical findings. Directions for future research are often indicated and, where appropriate, recommendations for clinical practice are made.

In developing this volume, we have attempted to combine some of the strengths of an authored book with those of an edited one. Most of the chapters were written by a combination of editors, often with an additional outside person contributing to the chapter. By using this strategy we hoped to provide a concentrated treatment of each topic while maintaining stylistic consistency from one chapter to the next.

Several guidelines were used in selecting topics for the present work. First, we identified the events that seem most central to reproduction and thus likely to be experienced by many persons. Second, we wanted topics for which a significant amount of work on the psychological and social aspects had been done. Even with these guidelines, the list of possible topics went beyond the scope of the present work. Consequently, rather than to strive for comprehensiveness, we attempted to provide in-depth examination of certain key events in human reproduction.

Initially we wanted a balanced coverage of topics for both men and women; however, it soon became apparent that neither had there been much work done concerning reproductive events of men nor had the psychological response of men to reproductive events of their wives or female partners received much attention. So the chapters are oriented strongly to the reproductive events of women with a discussion of the psychological and social aspects of these events for men presented wherever possible.

We hope this book will serve as a text and resource volume for workers in human reproduction, sexuality, mental health, and medicine. Furthermore, we hope it advances the development of an overall orientation to the psychology of the reproductive life cycle.

## ACKNOWLEDGMENTS

We wish to thank a variety of persons, all of whom contributed significantly to the process of preparing this book. The reference department of the Atkins Library of the University of North Carolina at Charlotte deserves special mention for their continued professional assistance in obtaining the relevant literature: Dawn Hubbs, Marcia Duncan, Jay Whaley, Mozelle Scherger, Judy O'Dell, Carol Iglauer, Lorraine Penninger, Barbara Lisenby, and Carl Clark. We thank Jacob Christ and Barry McGough for reading drafts and for making helpful critical comments. Ronnie Moon and Moira Jack provided capable clerical and editorial assistance. Helen Brayce, Dee Malcolon, Patricia Tyson, and Theresa Guitierrez deserve our thanks for typing. We thank also Laura Moore, Deb Dellinger, Rene Pearce, Melody Wilder, and Michael Mulvaney for their capable help, and Patricia L. Cato and Douglas P. Warren for their patient assistance with the typed manuscript.

# An Introduction to the Critical Life Problem Approach to Human Reproduction

EVENTS IN THE REPRODUCTIVE CYCLE are part of adult life for most people. Conception, pregnancy, childbirth, and relating to a newborn are events that sometimes enrich, sometimes frustrate, and sometimes distress those experiencing them. Certainly they change the pattern of life for most people. Examining the psychological and social aspects of some of these events is the purpose of the present volume.

The reproductive dimension of human sexuality has received little attention from behavioral scientists. Instances of severe psychopathology occurring in relation to a particular reproductive event (e.g., childbirth) have been the major focus of discussions on psychosocial factors in this area. Often, discussion has centered on whether disturbances associated in time with a major reproductive event represent forms of psychopathology different from disturbances occurring at other times. At issue is whether the onset of major psychiatric disturbance is more likely at times of major reproductive transition, whether psychosocial or hormonal variables are primary causal factors since both sets are undergoing obvious changes, and whether treatment effectiveness parallels treatment effectiveness of disturbances occurring at other times.

Emphasis on cases of extreme disturbance has led to several conceptual and methodological limitations. Many of the often cited papers are based on series of cases of severely disturbed individuals. The data often consist of retrospective accounts or of the clinical record, including psychiatric observations and discussion of physical aspects of the case. Both of these sources are subject to significant biases either in terms of the recollection of patients and those around them or in terms of the interpretive biases of the clinician working with the patient.

This emphasis on cases of extreme psychiatric disturbance occurring in relation to a reproductive event also focuses attention on the individual in terms of potential biochemical factors, internal psychological conflicts, or perception of new role demands. The reproductive event (e.g., pregnancy) is thought of as a global occurrence. Psychiatric disturbance is seen, in part, as a response to this global event. Aspects of the behavioral responses of the people are not generally examined as a function of the range of specific variables subsumed under the global heading.

In the present volume, we have adopted a different perspective. Instead of focusing on cases of severe psychiatric disturbance occurring in relation to some reproductive event, we begin with an emphasis on the reproductive events themselves. We view them as critical life problems (Calhoun, Selby, & King, 1976) confronted by most people. Events like pregnancy and childbirth are seen as significant transitions for women and men. Some master the transitions with relative ease while others experience mild, moderate, or severe disturbance. The degree and duration of such disturbance would be expected to vary with the characteristics of the changes in physical functioning (e.g., a disabling pregnancy symptom), the nature and extent of new demands, as well as the psychological and social resources available to meet such demands.

Discussing pregnancy and childbirth in particular may help to clarify the critical life problem approach to understanding the psychology of reproductive events generally. Pregnancy and childbirth are, of course, actually comprised of a whole set of specific components, including the objective physical changes associated with conception, gestation, and parturition, the perception of these bodily changes by the pregnant woman and her husband or partner, the affective responses of both, and the thoughts, beliefs, and expectations of each concerning these events. Social changes encompass the relationship between the pregnant woman and her partner, as well as their relationships with friends and other family members, relationships with the health care professionals concerned with reproduction, and the demands and characteristics of the neonate. There are measurable differences in the extent to which each of these factors occurs in the pregnancy of a given individual or couple. Thus, the challenge posed to personal and social adjustment differs with each pregnancy. For example, a couple who strongly hold the cultural expectation of a glowing maternalism with a cuddly baby, if faced with a baby who is physically defective, may feel considerable disappointment, worry, or depression.

A person's responses to events like pregnancy and childbirth are in part determined by personal and social resources available when problems occur. Those with more meager resources or those in whom existing resources were already taxed by nonpregnancy demands would be expected to show greater dysfunction associated with comparable pregnancy events than persons having greater resources or persons whose existing resources were not so taxed.

The characteristics of the particular reproductive event, along with the availability of personal and social resources, affect the kind or degree of distress. For instance, for a woman who has a poor relationship with her husband and whose pregnancy is marked by severe nausea and vomiting, sexual distress and general dissatisfaction during pregnancy may be especially severe.

The critical life problems approach has several important implications for understanding the psychological aspects of reproductive events. The approach recognizes a continuum of distress. It begins with the assumption that the variables involved in the more common mild and moderate distress would be the same factors likely to be involved in more infrequent but extreme distress. Furthermore, the present approach encourages prospective studies, including normative descriptions of the psychological responses correlated with the different phases of each event within the reproductive life cycle. Such prospective studies can be more methodologically sound than the typical retrospective case study. The present framework, through the development of predictive indices of future distress, is also congruent with identification of high-risk groups. A basis for the development and evaluation of both preventive and treatment measures for psychological distress associated with the events is also suggested herein. Finally, the present framework extends the kind of theorizing and work begun on the psychological aspects of pregnancy (Bibring, 1959; Bibring et al., 1961; Bibring & Valenstein, 1976) to reproductive events generally. Such extension would encourage the integration of findings and hypotheses into a psychology of human reproduction.

In this book we have attempted to use the critical life problems approach to reproductive events. Existing work on the issues in pregnancy are discussed, including psychological changes in pregnancy, the value of prepared childbirth, and psychological responses to terminated pregnancy. Major events in the postdelivery period are examined, among them the psychological factors in postpartum reactions, implications of early parent-neonate interactions, reactions to preterm birth, and psychological impact of having a handicapped baby. Finally, changes in the reproductive system are discussed. These changes involve the psychological dimensions in controlling conception, as well as the psychological correlates of menopause and climacteric.

These events were selected because they seem central and because a reasonable amount of theory and research on each exists. Across all of these events, several trends emerge. Most of the work has been devoted to the psychological, psychiatric, and social functioning of women in relation to reproductive events, with limited discussion of their impact on men. As Parlee (1976) noted, most theorizing on childbirth emphasizes either the intrapsychic conflicts or the hormonal changes thought to occur within women at that time. Cognitive and interpersonal dimensions have received far less attention. Likewise, research on the psychology of men during these transitional periods is almost nonexistent. Each chapter attempts to reflect the current knowledge of the psychology of women and of men during reproductive events.

Through these chapters we present up-to-date information concerning the psychological changes associated with some events in the reproductive life cycle. An understanding of available knowledge is fundamental to providing good psychological assistance. As pointed out by Selby and Calhoun (1980), conveying accurate, personally relevant information about the problem situation to persons experiencing that situation can reduce uncertainty and facilitate a more positive approach. Though traditional therapies have not emphasized the role of factual information in treatment, the potential value of sound cognitive understanding has been highlighted with respect to sexual dysfunctions (Annon, 1974; Cherwick & Cherwick, 1971; Masters & Johnson, 1970), coping with surgery (Auerbach & Kilmann, 1977; Egbert et al., 1964; Schmitt & Woolridge, 1973), and coping with a handicapped child (Ehlers, 1966; Grossman, 1972; Stone, 1967). Within the realm of reproduction, the value of factual information has been stressed in prepared childbirth programs (Klusman, 1975). We believe the value extends to all of the events within the reproductive cycle.

Bringing together current knowledge concerning the psychological changes during particular reproductive events also allows for the formulation of treatment procedures specific to each event. Medical and psychological procedures and specialized resources can be better tailored to the problems and pitfalls associated with each major event, and particular recommendations are made within the book.

Traditional therapies for psychological disturbances associated with reproduction have been oriented to treatment rather than prevention. Psychoanalytically oriented therapists and theorists have long hoped that the dissemination of knowledge concerning intrapsychical events to individuals and care-giving institutions would assist in both preventing and treating psychological pathology, particularly that associated with childbearing and child-rearing. The authors noted above have demonstrated that in specific areas cognitive information can have a salutary effect on psychological response to reproductive events. We, however, suggest caution in predicting the demise of distress related to human reproduction even if massive programs of individual, public, and institutional education concerning reproduction are implemented. Indeed the critical life problem approach espoused in this volume suggests that just as individual responses to reproductive events are extremely variable and represent probabilities and not certainties, so treatment and prevention strategies which are based on probable responses must be individually variable to be most effective. Thus for one woman appropriate prevention of peripartum psychological distress may rest on the transmission of cognitive information concerning pregnancy, whereas for another, prevention may be best accomplished by an examination of that woman's relationship with her own mother.

We believe the present volume will advance the psychology of human reproduction as a field of study. Certainly, this area of living is vitally important to the psychological adjustment of most adults. Examining theory and research related to reproductive events would seem fundamental to the development of an overall understanding of the psychological adjustment of adults.

## REFERENCES

Annon, J. S. *The behavioral treatment of sexual problems. Vol. 1: Brief therapy.* Honolulu: Enabling Systems, 1974.

Auerbach, S. M., and Kilmann, P. R. Crisis intervention: A review of outcome research. *Psychological Bulletin,* 1977, *84,* 1189–1217.

Bibring, L. Some considerations of the psychological processes in pregnancy. *Psychoanalytic Study of the Child,* 1959, *14,* 113–121.

Bibring, L., Dwyer, F., Huntington, S., and Valenstein, A. A study of the psychological processes in pregnancy and of the earliest mother-child relationship: Part 1: Some propositions and comments. *Psychoanalytic Study of the Child,* 1961, *16,* 9–24.

Bibring, L., and Valenstein, A. Psychological aspects of pregnancy. *Clinical Obstetrics and Gynecology,* 1976, *19,* 357–371.

Calhoun, L. G., Selby, J. W., and King, H. E. *Dealing with crisis.* Englewood Cliffs: Prentice-Hall, 1976.

Cherwick, A. B., and Cherwick, B. The role of ignorance in sexual dysfunction. *Psychosomatics,* 1971, *12,* 235–244.

Egbert, L. D., Battit, G. E., Welch, C. E., and Bartlett, M. K. Reduction of postoperative pain by encouragement and instruction of patients. *New England Journal of Medicine,* 1964, *270,* 825–827.

Ehlers, W. H. *Mothers of retarded children.* Springfield: Charles C Thomas, 1966.

Grossman, F. K. *Brothers and sisters of retarded children.* Syracuse: Syracuse University Press, 1972.

Klusman, L. E. Reduction of pain in childbirth by the alleviation of anxiety during pregnancy. *Journal of Consulting and Clinical Psychology,* 1975, *43,* 162–165.

Masters, W. H., and Johnson, V. E. *Human sexual inadequacy.* Boston: Little, Brown, 1970.

Parlee, M. B. Social factors in the psychology of menstruation, birth, and menopause. *Primary Care,* 1976, *3,* 477–490.

Schmitt, F. E., and Woolridge, P. J. Psychological preparation of surgical patients. *Nursing Research,* 1973, *22,* 108–116.

Selby, J. W., and Calhoun, L. G. The psychodidactic element of psychological intervention: an undervalued and underdeveloped treatment tool. *Professional Psychology,* in press.

Stone, N. D. Family factors in willingness to place the mongoloid child. *American Journal of Mental Deficiency,* 1967, *72,* 16–20.

# PART I

## PREGNANCY

# Chapter 1

# Psychological Changes in Pregnancy

PREGNANCY IS A MAJOR EVENT within human reproduction. Although considerable scientific attention has been devoted to the physiological processes of pregnancy, little systematic research has addressed the psychological or interpersonal changes accompanying this state. The bulk of the literature regarding psychological reactions to pregnancy consists of individual case studies or poorly controlled retrospective studies. There exist few prospective studies regarding psychological reactions to pregnancy; therefore, any formulations regarding reactions to pregnancy must be considered tentative. This chapter will examine some available research data and current theorizing relevant to the psychological and social aspects of pregnancy.

Deutsch (1945) was one of the first to focus on the psychology of women, including their reactions to pregnancy. She noted the tremendous physiological changes that occur with pregnancy but believed that psychological factors exaggerated symptoms such as nausea, lack of appetite, ravenous hunger, or food cravings. Thus, although not ignoring the modified gastric secretions, Deutsch did view excessive nausea or vomiting as being related to conflicts about the pregnancy. On the other hand, she viewed the normal pregnancy as being accompanied by some physical problems (nausea, vomiting, gastrointestinal symptoms) and some emotional upheaval and lability.

Deutsch described pregnancy as a time of turning inward. She regarded this process as the woman's devoting her psychic energies to the fetus and to her fantasies about it as an object outside herself. Thus, there appear to be several psychological stages related to acceptance of the fetus. First, the mother must acknowledge and accept a being who exists within her body, causing some discomfort, hormonal and endocrinological changes, as well as a change in her physical appearance. After initial acceptance, fantasies about the fetus and its future form the initial stage of motherly love, and the pregnant woman becomes less emotionally involved with external events and surroundings. The *quickening,* or initial movement, of the fetus promotes an intensification of the mother-child relationship as the mother has "proof" of a living being within her whom she physically experiences. She can demonstrate its living presence to everyone and engage in some sort of an active relationship with the fetus as it kicks and moves. This also heralds the beginning of the next psychological stage for the mother: preparation for relinquishing the fetus to the outer world.

Deutsch thought that the pregnant woman's identification with her own mother, as well as with the fetus she is carrying, is critically related to the capacity for motherhood. If major conflicts exist involving these identifications severe difficulties arise. If the woman cannot identify with the fetus she carries she may become rejecting of it. This may increase the difficulty of the pregnancy and may contribute to spontaneous or habitual abortion.

The process and quality of identification with her own mother may give rise to difficulties for the pregnant woman and her child. In Deutsch's view, it is through a review and revising of the pregnant woman's relationship with her own mother that she is no longer "the child of the mother, but the mother of the child" (p. 145). Thus, the pregnant woman is able to include positive aspects of her own mother into her newly emerging self-concept as a mother.

Finally, Deutsch emphasized the relationship of the woman with her husband as having significant effects on the woman's pregnancy, feelings for the unborn child, and perhaps ability to carry the child to term. She postulated that negative feelings toward the husband can be directed toward the product of their union and can have long-term effects on the mother-child relationship. Furthermore, a pregnancy in which the husband is not available to provide emotional and physical support can be a very difficult one.

Although largely based on the psychoanalysis of women with psychopathology, these theories may be useful in understanding the psychology of pregnancy.

Bibring and her associates (Bibring, 1959; Bibring et al., 1961a, b; Bibring & Valenstein, 1976) were intrigued with the high percentage of obstetrical patients at a prenatal clinic who were viewed as having psychiatric problems. Although Deutsch (1945) had suggested that irrational behavior may increase during pregnancy, Bibring et al. (1961a, b) were astounded at the frequency with which psychiatric interviews revealed the presence of depression, anxiety, and paranoid mechanisms.

More surprising, these women responded dramatically to minimal therapeutic support and never became seriously disturbed. Following delivery the majority of the women found pregnancy, delivery, and motherhood quite within their capabilities. The consistency of these findings led Bibring et al. (1961b) to hypothesize that this picture is reflective of the condition of pregnancy rather than of the specific pathology of the women referred to them.

Bibring and her colleagues conceptualized pregnancy as a period of profound psychological as well as somatic changes. Like puberty and menopause, pregnancy is a developmental task that requires both adjustment and the resolution of conflicts from earlier developmental phases. Bibring's conceptualization of pregnancy as a developmental stage or task is strikingly similar to Erikson's (1963) formulations regarding personality development. Erikson postulated that there are eight stages or crises, each having a specific developmental task necessary for the formulation of a healthy, mature personality. Pregnancy is a stage in which the personality is in disequilibrium and new tasks, acceptance of a feminine role, and reformulation of relationships with important others are accomplished. The crisis of pregnancy may result in maturation or, under unfavorable conditions, it may result in instances of dysfunctional femininity and motherhood. In either event the outcome of the crisis will profoundly affect the mother-child relationship.

## ATTITUDES TOWARD PREGNANCY

Often the reaction of a woman to the news of her pregnancy does not appear to be the joyous excitement commonly portrayed in folklore. The literature and clinical experience suggests that many women are unhappy or ambivalent about the news of pregnancy.

Leifer (1977) found that approximately one-half of the 19 women she studied were ambivalent or negative about the pregnancy; however, by the end of the pregnancy moderately positive attitudes prevailed. Winokur and Werhoff (1956) noted similar changes in acceptance as the pregnancy progressed. Of the 30 women in their study who reported not wanting the baby initially, only 2 indicated that they did not want the child during the third trimester.

A woman's attitude toward her pregnancy especially with regard to acceptance does not appear to be directly related to whether or not the pregnancy was planned. In fact, the incidence of unplanned pregnancies appears quite high in view of the numerous contraceptives available. Wenner, Cohen, Weigert, Kvarnes, Ohaneson, and Fearing (1969) reported that 50% of the 52 women they interviewed had unplanned pregnancies. Eighteen women accepted the unplanned pregnancy while eight never accepted it. Morris (1963), relying on a sample of 34 women, noted that 19, as opposed to only 15 husbands, reported having planned pregnancies. Twenty-four of both husbands and wives said that they were pleased with the pregnancy. Netter (1977) discussed findings that suggest that unplanned pregnancies in women who have lost a child are much wanted, whereas unplanned pregnancies in newlywed or higher socioeconomic status women may be resented.

Women who had no children were found to be more likely to be pleased with a pregnancy than were women with children (Winokur & Werhoff, 1956). Sears, Maccoby, and Levin (1957) noted that of 379 women studied almost twice as many recalled being happy with the first pregnancy as compared to later pregnancies. Gordon et al. (1965) found that 80% of the women in his study were happy about their first one or two children but only 31% were happy about the fourth or more. Differences in acceptance were also correlated with spacing between pregnancies. Fifty-two percent of those women with children coming 55 months apart were delighted with the pregnancy as opposed to only 9% of the mothers whose children were born less than 21 months apart (Sears, Maccoby, & Levin, 1957).

In summary it appears that the initial reaction of many women (50–60%) to the news of a pregnancy is rejection or ambivalence. For these women acceptance of the pregnancy appears to be a gradual process, and by the third trimester most women view their pregnancy positively. Acceptance of a pregnancy is not directly correlated with whether or not it was planned. Unplanned pregnancies are frequent and are likely to be accepted by most women. A more salient factor affecting acceptance appears to be whether the woman already has children. First pregnancies are the most likely to be wanted. For the woman who has had children previously, the longer the space between children, the more likely the pregnancy is to be welcome.

## EMOTIONAL FACTORS

A special part of pregnancy adjustment is thought to be a reorientation of the pregnant woman toward her own mother. The majority of support comes from psychodynamic clinical studies (Bibring, 1959). Despres (1937), in a study of 100 primiparas, found that a close relationship with mother, happy home life, sexual and social compatibility with husband, and economic security significantly distinguished women with favorable attitudes toward pregnancy from those with unfavorable attitudes. Newton (1955) interviewed 123 women postpartum and found intercorrelations between feelings toward menstruation, sex, childbirth, breastfeeding, infant care, and the desirability of being a woman. A positive attitude in one area was related to a positive attitude in another. These studies suffer from serious methodological problems, but some of their hypotheses find support in later studies.

Zemlick and Watson (1953) studied 15 women to determine whether acceptance-rejection of pregnancy, degree of anxiety, or tendency toward somatization could be used to predict adjustment during pregnancy, delivery, and the immediate postpartum period. Women were seen between the second and the fifth lunar month of pregnancy, six weeks prior to delivery, and again six weeks postdelivery. The instruments used as predictors were the Thematic Apperception Test (TAT), the McFarland-Seitz Psychosomatic Inventory, and the ZAR Pregnancy Attitude Scale. The TAT allows the subject to project personality characteristics, as well as his or her wishes and fears, through the telling of stories in response to a relatively neutral stimulus card. Ten cards were used in this study. The stories told by each woman were then rated by three independent judges on an eight-point scale for anxiety. The Psychosomatic Inventory is a standardized questionnaire that covers various symptoms. The Pregnancy Attitude Scale is a questionnaire designed to measure the subjective attitudes of women concerning pregnancy and motherhood by having the subject complete or rate a statement on a six-point continuum from "always" to "never." The criterion measures were the ratings of physical and emotional symptoms during office visits, the time in labor, ratings of the woman's adjustment in labor, and ratings of the mother-baby interaction.

Anxiety as derived from the TAT was found to be inversely related to adjustment in pregnancy and delivery but not related to mother-baby interaction. All predictor measures were found to be positively correlated with independent clinical ratings of prenatal adjustment and delivery. Surprisingly, attitudes of rejection of the pregnancy were found to be inversely related to high ratings of mother-baby interaction. Zemlick and Watson (1953) postulated that the extremes of those behaviors rated positively by an anthropologist in observing mother-baby interactions were in fact not positive but "over-protective." They theorized that those mothers who evidenced rejection or ambivalence prepartum, having both psychological and somatic symptoms, repressed their negative feelings after the birth of the baby and became "over-protective."

Another plausible explanation for these results may be that the scores on the Pregnancy Attitude Scale actually represented the difficulties experienced physically and emotionally during the pregnancy. Once the pregnancy ended, the woman experienced relief. Ratings after delivery were less confounded by aspects of the pregnancy and were directly related to the baby. Some support for this hypothesis is found in the fact that three of the women in the "rejecting/over-protective" group either had been sterile or had had a previous miscarriage, experiences that probably increased anxiety during the pregnancy. Later studies (Zuckerman et al., 1963) have found significant positive correlations between anxiety and somatic symptoms.

Davids and Holden (1970) utilized the Parental Attitude Research Instrument (PARI) to assess maternal attitudes toward family life and childrearing during pregnancy (third trimester) and at eight months postpartum. Factor analysis of the six subscales of the PARI showed two main factors, one termed "hostility" and the other, "control." Ratings on several personality characteristics such as depression and anxiety were made by the examining psychologist during an interview eight months postpartum. Independent ratings of the mother and mother-child interaction were also made eight months postpartum.

Forty-two women of diverse racial, social, and cultural backgrounds were evaluated; however, for the postpartum assessment maternal personality ratings were available for only 27 of the original group. PARI scores during pregnancy were significantly associated with those after delivery, as well as with the personality ratings. Women whose PARI scores were high on the hostility factor were high on anxiety and depression. A negative association between high hostility scores and favorableness of personality evaluations was noted. Similar associations for the control factor were found, but the only significant association was a positive one for the depression rating.

Comparison of PARI scores during pregnancy and the follow-up personality ratings revealed a statistically significant positive correlation of undesirable family and childrearing attitudes in pregnancy with anxiety and depression. A negative association was found for undesirable attitudes and favorable mother-child interaction ratings. Thus, there is statistical evidence of consistency in attitudes acknowledged during pregnancy and after the child was eight months old. These findings are in contrast to those of Zemlick and Watson (1953), who found a positive correlation between a rejecting attitude toward the child during pregnancy and positive ratings of mother-infant interaction.

The factors affecting maternal attitudes during pregnancy and after delivery are numerous and complex. To date, the literature on pregnancy has failed to produce stable and robust findings on many of the variables that have been hypothesized to affect the woman (depression, anxiety, happiness, physical changes, etc.). Until more sophisticated studies controlling larger numbers of variables are conducted, attempts to account for stability or inconsistencies in maternal attitudes must be considered speculative.

## BODY IMAGE

The concept of body image refers to the mental picture a person has of his or her body. It is a perception based on past and current experiences and encompasses height, weight, facial features, voice, etc. Since current experiences and perceptions may affect body image, it is a dynamic concept rather than a static one. Consequently, it seems reasonable to expect that body image changes during pregnancy. In studying this phenomenon, investigators have adopted somewhat different strategies of measuring body image.

Fisher and Cleveland (1958) developed a content scoring system of the Rorschach test based on two aspects of body image: barrier (B) and penetration (P). The Rorschach is a projective test designed to elicit unconscious thoughts and feelings. The subject is shown a series of 10 stimulus cards that look like inkblots and is asked to tell what he or she sees in each card. Thus, the subject free associates to an ambiguous and neutral stimulus and projects his or her own unconscious thoughts and feelings onto it. *Barrier* refers to responses on the Rorschach relating to the definiteness and strength of boundaries (e.g., knight in armor). *Penetration* refers to those responses implying vulnerability or weakness of boundaries (e.g., soft ice cream).

McConnell and Daston (1961) studied body image changes in 28 women during the third trimester and immediately postpartum. There were no unusual pregnancies or deliveries. Each person was seen twice during the eighth and ninth months of pregnancy and three days after delivery. At the initial meeting the women were interviewed; both the Rorschach and the Semantic Differential were administered. During the second session some women were able to complete only the Semantic Differential (due to discharge from the hospital). Attitude toward pregnancy, either positive or negative, was assessed independently by five psychologists examining the interviews.

The Semantic Differential was scored by computing mean scores on each of the three factors: evaluative, potency, and activity. Comparing self-evaluations by the subjects, the authors found a higher evaluation of the body after delivery than during pregnancy. During pregnancy the women viewed themselves as being in an unnatural condition and saw their bodies as ugly, misshapen, and devalued. The women viewed their bodies as less potent after delivery. This shift probably reflects the body changes taking place. For example, the body was described as "hard" and "thick" during the pregnancy but "soft" and "thin" after delivery.

The Rorschach protocols showed a statistically significant decrease in penetration scores after delivery. The authors hypothesized that pregnancy involves an intense emotional upheaval and that an individual may feel less integrated and more vulnerable during pregnancy. Fantasies of body boundary disruption may also arise as the mother anticipates the actual penetration of body boundaries during the birth experience. Following delivery, anxiety and fear become less intense and penetration scores decrease. Barrier scores reflected no change. McConnell and Daston (1961) suggested that the barrier concept refers to a more stable aspect of body image.

Attitude toward pregnancy, as judged from the interviews before childbirth, was compared with the three factors of the Semantic Differential obtained postpartum. The only significant findings concerned the evaluative factor. Women who viewed the pregnancy positively viewed their bodies positively during pregnancy but negatively postdelivery. Women who viewed pregnancy negatively viewed their bodies negatively during pregnancy but positively postdelivery.

The attitude measures (from the interviews) were compared with the Rorschach measures. Women with positive attitudes had higher barrier scores than those with negative attitudes.

McConnell and Daston (1961) theorized that their findings are conceptually compatible with Bibring's finding (1959, 1961a, b, 1976) that pregnant women seem to experience emotional disequilibrium without necessarily becoming psychiatrically disturbed. The findings with regard to P scores may reflect feelings of disequilibrium, while B scores may indicate no serious impairment of ego strength. Inferential support for this reasoning comes from comparing the scores of college students and schizophrenics with these pregnant women's scores. The women's B scores were approximately equal to those of a normative group of 200 college students, but their P scores were higher; the P scores were more like those of the schizophrenics (Fisher & Cleveland, 1958).

Tolor and Digrazia (1976) attempted to study body image changes of pregnant women as reflected in their human figure drawings. The drawing is assumed to portray the body image of the respondent and to contain both conscious and unconscious perceptions of the self. Drawings were obtained from five groups of women: 54 women in the first trimester of pregnancy; 51 in the second; 56 in the third; 55 at six weeks postpartum; and a control group of 76 women with gynecological problems. (The women in these five groups were white and married, with a mean age of 27.6 years and a mean educational level of 13.6 years.) The women were asked to draw "a whole woman" by the nurse in the obstetrician's office. The drawings were scored by three raters on nine forced-choice scales, an example being "dressed" versus "not dressed." Final judgment required two out of three ratings to agree. Perfect agreement was obtained by the three raters on 79% of the drawings. The poorest reliability was on "relatively well differentiated" versus "relatively poorly differentiated," which was agreed upon 64% of the time.

Tolor and Digrazia (1976) found no differences across the trimesters. Combining the three trimester groups and comparing them to the postpartum group also failed to show significant results on the majority of comparisons. The only finding was that the postpartum group had more shading in the drawings; this was assumed to indicate increased anxiety. However, the total number of comparisons would produce at least one chance finding, and the authors attributed this finding to chance.

In comparing the pregnant women to the women with gynecological problems, the authors noted some interesting differences. Pregnant women more frequently drew nude figures, sexual organs, and distorted figures; they were therefore assumed to be more preoccupied with their bodies. Their drawings suggested sexual preoccupation or concerns, as well as changes or distortions in body image.

The lack of findings regarding stages of pregnancy are surprising in view of the body changes in pregnancy. The most reasonable explanation is that the criterion measures, i.e., a figure drawing of a woman, rated on nine scales, were crude and insensitive. The research on projective drawings suggests equivocal validity and reliability for the instruments. Furthermore, the nine scales used for rating may not have been the best. The failure to follow the same women over the three trimesters was certainly a limitation of this study. It is possible that there were differences between groups on factors other than stage of pregnancy, which may be an additional explanation for the lack of findings regarding trimesters.

Uddenberg and Hakanson (1972) utilized aniseikonic lenses to study body perceptions during pregnancy. These lenses are designed to distort objects viewed through them. The amount of distortion varies among individuals; however, several studies (Fisher & Rechter, 1970; Wittreich and Radcliffe, 1955) have demonstrated that psychological factors such as anxiety may decrease the distortions. For example, Fisher and Rechter (1970) showed that the more imminent menstruation, the less distorted the pelvis was perceived. Pregnancy, like menstruation, is a part of reproduction and is generally associated with the pelvis; therefore, Uddenberg and Hakanson (1972) hypothesized that the greater the number of conflicts associated with the pregnancy, the less likely a woman would be to perceive her own pelvis as distorted when viewed through aniseikonic glasses.

Forty-five randomly selected primigravidas between the fourteenth and the nineteenth week of pregnancy were interviewed. Attitudes toward pregnancy, mental disturbances (tension, anxiety, depression), sexual dysfunction, and relationships with others were explored. The aniseikonic body perception was then studied by having each woman look at herself in a mirror and rank the relative degree of distortion of each body region (head, chest, abdomen, arms, pelvis, and legs). The results indicated that women reporting many symptoms before the pregnancy, as well as during the pregnancy, perceived the pelvis as relatively less distorted. Significant findings were also noted with regard to sexual conflicts and a less distorted perception of the pelvis. No significant associations were noted for the women's attitude toward pregnancy, marital status, or education. The authors viewed these findings as the result of a perceptual defense on the part of the women. That is, the woman who is conflicted about her pregnancy and who has mental symptoms such as anxiety or depression, or the woman who has sexual difficulties, will avoid attending to the pelvis, the body area associated with these conflicts, and thus will experience less distortion.

## SEXUALITY AND COITUS DURING PREGNANCY

Landis, Poffenberger, and Poffenberger (1950) conducted one of the first studies on sexuality during pregnancy. Anonymous questionnaires were distributed to 228 couples who had recently gone through their first pregnancy. Separate questionnaires for both husband and wife were obtained for 212 couples whose first child was not more than two and one-half years old. More than half of the wives and husbands (58%) felt that their sexual adjustment was not affected by the pregnancy. Almost one-fourth found the effect unfavorable; almost one-fifth found it favorable. Interestingly, the group that saw the pregnancy as improving sexual adjustment tended to have had poor adjustment before conception.

Both husbands and wives reported a decrease in sexual desire over the course of the pregnancy. Seventy-nine percent of the wives reported less desire during the third three months whereas 64% of the husbands reported less desire. Only 20% of the husbands and 16% of the wives reported the same desire during this period of time. Looking at the similarity of responses, Landis and associates (1950) hypothesized that psychological rather than physiological factors were responsible for this decrease. A consistent tendency appeared for couples who reported increased desire to rate themselves as happier than those couples whose desire remained the same or diminished during pregnancy.

Following the birth the general level of sexual desire was somewhat lower than it was before pregnancy. Fear of another pregnancy interfered with sexual adjustment, and wives who had confidence in their contraceptive had better sexual adjustment.

Falicov (1973) studied 19 primigravidas with regard to sexual adjustment during pregnancy and postpartum. Subjects were chosen in serial order if they met the following criteria: living with husband; pregnancy planned; no psychiatric or physical difficulties; no previous miscarriages, abortions, or gynecological complications; white; and middle-class. This sample was similar to that selected by Landis et al. (1950).

Each woman was interviewed five times: first, second, and third trimesters, postdelivery, and six to eight weeks postpartum. The investigator, relying on the interviews, rated (1) frequency of coitus, (2) degree of sexual desire, and (3) feelings of eroticism and satisfaction on a five-point scale. (The co-investigator also rated, and 80% agreement was obtained.)

Eighteen of the 19 had a decrease on all three factors during the first trimester. Fatigue, sleepiness, and nausea were noted, as were fears of harming the fetus (10 women), although the fears were recognized as unreasonable. The second trimester saw a rise in frequency of coitus and in sexual satisfaction relative to the first trimester scores although below prepregnancy levels. Desire remained at the same level as during the first trimester, with necessitated changes in position reported as a hindrance. Fears of harming the fetus continued for nine of the women. By the third trimester fluctuations in desire were frequent (seven), but one-half of the women who reported tension earlier in the pregnancy felt more relaxed, and sex was more enjoyable. Interestingly, the fears of harm had decreased. During the last two months frequency dropped dramatically, with 15 of the women reporting no intercourse.

Seven weeks postpartum intercourse was less frequent than it had been prepartum for 10 of the 19 couples. Fatigue and tension appeared to be the major factors responsible for the decrease, as desire and eroticism increased to previous levels. (Nine of the women reported an increased capacity for arousal and orgasm).

Two of these findings are inconsistent with those reported by Masters and Johnson (1966). Masters and Johnson reported (1) an increase in interest in the second trimester above prepregnancy levels and (2) a return to prepregnancy levels of interest and frequency of coital activity for all subjects within six to eight weeks postdelivery. These differences may reflect differences in the samples with regard to parity. The Masters and Johnson sample was largely multiparous.

Solberg, Butler, and Wagner (1973) interviewed 260 women postpartum concerning sexual behavior in pregnancy. Their sample was largely married (98%), multigravida (65%), white (93%), and relatively well educated. Male medical students, using a highly structured interview technique, served as interviewers. The pregnancy was divided into five stages: first trimester, second trimester, seventh month, eighth month, and ninth month. The year before becoming pregnant served as a baseline. Only women with full-term deliveries were included in this study.

Significant differences in frequency of coitus were reported between each stage, with the mean coital frequency for those women continuing to engage in coitus decreasing in a linear fashion. Coital frequency at all stages was independent of race, religious preference, educational level, negative feelings about pregnancy, or whether or not the pregnancy was planned. No association between coitus and previous pregnancies was noted. The index most associated with frequency was the level of sexual interest during pregnancy as compared with the level of the woman's interest before pregnancy. Those reporting a decrease in interest had lower frequency of intercourse than those whose interest remained the same or increased. This relationship did not hold for the ninth month of pregnancy.

Solberg et al. (1973) examined the reasons given by the women for the change in sexual behavior during pregnancy. Forty-six percent cited physical discomfort; fear of injuring the baby was noted by 27%; loss of interest, by 23%; and awkwardness, by 17%. Recommendations by a physician was noted by 8% of the women; 4% cited a loss of physical attractiveness; and 16% gave various other reasons. In contrast to the Masters and Johnson (1966) findings, the Solberg study indicated that women who received instructions to abstain from intercourse for two to eight weeks before the due date were significantly less sexually active than the other women during the ninth month of pregnancy but during no other time period.

Morris (1975), in a study of 900 pregnant and nonpregnant women in Thailand, found results similar to those of Solberg et al. (1973) in spite of a dramatically different methodology. Morris obtained data in a cross-sectional survey conducted by a specially trained public health nurse. Each woman was interviewed concerning her sexual behavior during the week before the interview. In order to compare the sexual behavior of the pregnant women (13% of the sample) and the nonpregnant women, Morris excluded women whose husbands were absent during the week in question and women who were menstruating. The responses of the remaining 490 nonpregnant women were compared with those of the 110 pregnant women. The periods of pregnancy were the same as those in the Solberg study: first trimester, second trimester, seventh, eighth, and ninth months of gestation.

The results showed a consistent downward trend in sexual activity as pregnancy progressed; however, the difference in sexual activity between the two groups was not statistically significant until the seventh month. The difference remained significant across the eighth- and ninth-month groups. Although a decline in sexual behavior as the pregnancy progressed confirmed the reports of Solberg et al. (1973), in the Morris (1975) study the slope of the decline in frequency is not linear but increases in the last trimester compared to the first two. In contrast, the degree of abstinence began to rise significantly in the second trimester in the Morris study, with the increase appearing linear. In the Solberg et al. study the rise in abstinence was delayed until the third trimester. The only reason given for the decline in sexual behavior by the Thai women was the pregnancy.

Both Solberg et al. (1973) and Morris (1975) noted that there is much individual variation in sexual behavior during pregnancy. Furthermore, they noted that cultural norms and even medical advice often discourage intercourse during pregnancy. In spite of these external factors, Solberg et al. suggested a biological basis for the decrease in frequency of intercourse during pregnancy and Morris argued that the cross-cultural consistency of the pattern lends strength to that hypothesis.

Tolor and Digrazia (1976) studied 216 women in various stages of pregnancy (first trimester, 54; second trimester, 51; and third trimester, 56) and at six weeks postpartum (55). The group was largely white (98%), married (99%), and well educated (a mean of 13.6 years of education), and most of the pregnancies were planned (61%). The physicians following these women placed no restrictions on sexual activity from conception until delivery unless medical complications occurred. Intercourse was prohibited during the first four weeks postpartum, after which the women were advised to consult their own comfort and preferences to determine frequency of sexual intercourse. Each woman was interviewed and responded to three questionnaires. One questionnaire obtained demographic data, another obtained information about sexual behavior, and the third was a 15-item attitude toward sex scale (Tolor, Rice, & Lanctot, 1975).

The results were consistent with those obtained in previous research in the area. Significant differences in desire for sexual activity across all four groups of women were observed. The desire for intercourse declined over the course of pregnancy but increased postpartum. The actual frequency of sexual behavior followed this pattern as well; however, the most pronounced decline in frequency occurred in the third trimester. (Almost one-third of the women in the third trimester reported no intercourse during this period.) Although first and second trimester women reported being satisfied with the rate of sexual activity, the third trimester women were less satisfied and preferred relatively less activity. The postpartum group reported more satisfaction, but 31% preferred more intercourse.

Studies conducted in the area of sexual behavior and sexual interest during pregnancy note wide individual variations but point to a pattern of declining interest and activity especially during the third trimester. Several authors have suggested biological factors (Morris, 1975; Solberg et al., 1973) in addition to cultural influences; however, these are only tentative hypotheses.

Coitus during pregnancy is frequently prohibited by physicians, and sexual intercourse during pregnancy has been cited as a possible cause of a variety of physical problems, including premature labor, miscarriage, and childhood epilepsy (Mann & Cunningham, 1972). A variety of studies have been conducted on the relationship between sexual behavior and sexual responses during pregnancy and potential physical abnormalities.

Pugh and Fernandez (1953) interviewed 500 women postpartum asking the last date of intercourse before delivery. The mean number of days to delivery following intercourse was 52, with the median being 28 days. The cases were then classified into three groups: complications related to coitus, complications unrelated to coitus, and no complications. Their study demonstrated no relationship between complications of late pregnancy or complications of delivery and coitus during pregnancy.

Goodlin, Keller, and Raffin (1971) interviewed a total of 200 women: 77% reported sexual orgasm during the second and third trimesters of pregnancy. Of the sample, 100 were interviewed during the second and third trimesters and 100 were interviewed postdelivery. Fifty women were chosen to be in the study because they had delivered prematurely; the 50 full-term controls were matched on age, social class, parity, and race. The 100 women who had delivered were then compared with regard to sexual activity.

Goodlin et al. found that the reported incidence of orgasm after 32 weeks was significantly higher in women who delivered prematurely (50%) than in those who delivered at term (20%). Twenty-six percent of the women delivering prematurely reported having achieved orgasm within 50 hours of labor compared to only 4% of the full-term group. Goodlin et al. noted that the full-term gravidas reported that orgasm sometimes caused lower abdominal discomfort or painful uterine contractions.

Grudzinskas, Watson, and Chard, (1979) reported in a study of 70 primiparous women that fetal distress (as measured by an Apgar score lower than 6 at one minute and meconium staining of the amniotic fluid) was more common when coitus occurred in the four weeks prior to delivery than when it did not. Naeye (1979) reports data gathered from 26,886 pregnancies over a 7 year period ending in 1966. The frequency of amniotic fluid infections was significantly greater in mothers who reported coitus once or more per week during the month before delivery compared to those women who reported no coitus. In addition, in the group with coitus the mortality of infected infants was nearly 5 times greater (11.0%) than that of the infected infants (2.4%) when there was no coitus reported. Finally, the frequencies of several other measures of fetal distress (low Apgar scores, neonatal respiratory distress, and hyperbilirubinemia) were nearly doubled when mothers reported coitus. The reasons for these differences are not understood but the possibility of increased bacterial penetration through the cervical os because of coitus seems plausible. Whether improved genital hygiene and/or the use of condoms or diaphragms can reduce fetal risk is as yet unknown.

Although the Goodlin study has not yet been replicated, its findings regarding uterine contractions have been noted by others (Masters & Johnson, 1966; Slate, 1970.) These authors, however, cautioned that the manner in which coitus may initiate or contribute to premature delivery or abortion is little understood and needs further investigation. These and other investigators (Mann & Cunningham, 1972; Neubardt, 1973; Parker, 1974) all have stressed that sexuality is a means of communication between marital partners. Thus, blanket prohibition of intercourse during the late months of pregnancy may ignore the woman's desire for sexual expression and may severely disrupt her relationship with her mate. Mann and Cunningham (1972) advised no limitation of sexual activities during a normally progressing pregnancy. Vaginal bleeding, ruptured membranes, or a ripe cervix all require medical consultation and are probable cause for limiting sexual activities. They further noted that women with a history of premature labor without obvious cause might benefit if intercourse were proscribed in light of the findings of Goodlin et al. (1971). Finally, Neubardt (1973) recommended that two aspects of sexuality during pregnancy should be understood by the pregnant woman. First, fluctuations in sexual interest, especially as the pregnancy progresses, are typical and are not a reason for concern because these fluctuations will not continue postpartum. Second, the woman needs reassurance regarding the relative protection of the fetus in the amniotic sac so that she and her mate will be free to find the position that is most comfortable for them in late pregnancy.

In summary, the research available suggests that the effects of pregnancy on a woman's sexual interest and activity are most pronounced during the third trimester. Fluctuations in sexual interest occur throughout pregnancy and a significant decrease in interest as well as sexual activity is typical during the third trimester. The research to date does not allow a delineation of the factors that might be responsible for this change although biological, psychological, and interpersonal influences have been hypothesized.

## EMOTIONAL CHANGES ACCOMPANYING PREGNANCY

Changes in mood or emotions during the nine months of pregnancy have been frequently cited in the clinical literature (Leifer, 1977). Coleman (1969) described intense feelings and mood changes during all three trimesters of pregnancy. He also noted that increased anxiety, fear of death, and fear of catastrophes were frequently mentioned by the six women in his study. Bushnell (1961) noted depression in 47 out of 55 cases; he viewed the degree of depression as so severe that amphetamines were prescribed. Tobin (1957) compared pregnant women with nonpregnant controls and noted that the "blues," crying, and irritability were significantly more prevalent in the pregnant group. In fact, 84% of the pregnant women reported having the blues.

Jarrahi-Zadeh, Kane, Van de Castle, Lachenbruch, and Ewing (1969) studied mood and mental functioning in the third trimester. Eighty-six women were evaluated during pregnancy and again postpartum. Insomnia (55%), mood lability (43%), and worry (40%) occurred more frequently during pregnancy. Multiparas complained of depression significantly more often during pregnancy and postpartum evaluations than did primiparas. Mood changes and fogginess in the postpartum period were also noted significantly more often by multiparas.

Kane, Harman, Keeler, and Ewing (1968) noted considerable subjective distress in 137 obstetrical patients. Sixty-four percent of the women told of feeling worse than usual during the pregnancy. The authors reported that 64% of the women appeared anxious and/or depressed and had cognitive dysfunction (by observation); however, objective test data did not strongly support these findings.

Nott, Franklin, Armitage, and Gelder (1976) evaluated 27 women two months before delivery on three measures of emotional upset or disturbance. The results from all three measures (a mood scale, a rating scale for symptoms related to the "maternity blues" syndrome, and a measure of symptoms of affective disorders) were supportive of findings from previous studies. A depressed mood and crying spells were observed for every woman in the study. Lability in mood and increased emotional responsiveness were frequently noted, as were lethargy and poor concentration. The Nott study concluded that it is erroneous to think in terms of the presence or absence of emotional disturbance, or the blues syndrome; rather, there appears to be a continuum of disturbance in all women around the time of delivery. The authors also concluded that a major difficulty in obtaining consistent prevalence rates of the blues may be the different methods of assessment (behavioral observation, clinical diagnosis, or scales of emotional disturbance).

To summarize, the most frequent emotional changes occurring through pregnancy appear to be depression, lability of mood, and increased emotional responsiveness. Symptoms of crying, irritability, insomnia, lethargy, and difficulty in concentration are also frequently noted. These changes are present in the majority of women; however, relatively few women become so distressed that their responses on mood and symptom scales indicate a significant degree of emotional disturbance.

## DEPENDENCY

Several authors have noted increased dependency, both emotional and physical, in pregnant women (Caplan, 1957; Liebenberg, 1969; Roehner, 1976). The majority of studies have not explained the types of behavior and/or emotional change that they have studied. Wenner et al. (1969) described an increased "mature" dependency during pregnancy related to communication of needs, seeking of assistance from appropriate people, acceptance of assistance, and recognition that the helper may have limitations (acceptance of partial gratification). The Wenner study concluded that the physical changes in pregnancy, as well as emotional changes, increase the dependency needs of the pregnant woman. All women in this study manifested a need for greater attention, reassurance that help was available, and a demonstration of interest and involvement on the part of friends and family.

A more systematic evaluation of dependency utilized an indirect measure: the wish to be held. Hollender and McGehee (1974) hypothesized that there would be an increased need to be held with pregnancy because of increased dependency, affiliative, or security needs. They studied 25 black and 25 white pregnant women, with an average age of 22 years. There were 17 single women in the study, 14 of them being black. Although this was the first pregnancy for most, the group was not homogeneous for parity. Twenty-three women reported an increased wish to be held with the pregnancy. The feelings of 19 women were unchanged and 8 women experienced a decrease in the wish to be held. Thus, more than half of the women noted a change during pregnancy in their wish to be held and of this group, three-fourths experienced an increase. There were no differences between primiparous and multiparous women. The authors concluded that pregnancy causes greater need for closeness, security, and succor.

## ANXIETY IN PREGNANCY

Grimm (1967) administered a short battery of projective tests to determine whether there are differences in the degree of "psychological tension" or anxiety over the 40-week course of pregnancy. She studied normal women divided into three groups: last half first trimester, first half third trimester, and second half third trimester. The women in each group were matched with respect to parity, race, marital status, age, education, religion, cultural background, and previous obstetric complications. The methodology was designed to avoid the contaminating effects of memory on the psychological tests.

Responses to three cards of the TAT were analyzed to determine tension or anxiety. The stories told by the women were scored with themes of injury, violence, aggression, or death being considered high on anxiety or tension. A greater number of women seen during the last half of the third trimester obtained scores indicative of disturbance, i.e., the tension index rose in the first half of the third trimester.

Lubin, Gardener, and Roth (1975) attempted to obtain baseline data concerning the natural history of a pregnancy. Their sample consisted of 93 white, middle-class women who had a mean educational level of 14 years and were married to medical students, interns, and residents. The women were divided into three groups: "no previous pregnancies," "previous live birth and no terminated pregnancy," and "previous live birth and previous terminated pregnancy." The Menstrual History Questionnaire (a frequency and severity of complaint instrument), the Anxiety Adjective Checklist (AACL, a self-administered checklist), the Depression Anxiety Checklist (DACL, a self-administered adjective checklist), the Symptom Checklist (SCL, a checklist of symptoms and complaints), and the IPAT Anxiety Scale Questionnaire (a self-report anxiety measure) were administered. The last four measures were administered during the second and third trimesters.

Seven two-way analyses of variance were performed, one for each measurement variable (AACL, DACL, SCL, and four IPAT scores). There was a significant difference in anxiety as measured by the AACL over trimesters, with anxiety during the second trimester being significantly lower. The authors noted that these findings coincided with many descriptions of anxiety over trimesters. The Symptom Checklist produced no significant differences over trimesters for all groups; however, the "previous live birth and previous terminated pregnancy" group did show a significant rise in somatic complaints during the second trimester, as well as a trend indicating greater depression (DACL). The authors postulated that these differences might reflect previous problems with pregnancy. Neither the DACL nor the IPAT showed significant differences over trimesters. Correlational analyses found significant positive relationships between somatic symptoms and anxiety and between history of menstrual complaints and somatic symptoms, along with a negative correlation between education and overt anxiety. The results confirmed the findings of an earlier study (Zuckerman et al., 1963) that had discovered that anxiety and somatic complaints are significantly correlated during pregnancy. Furthermore, it confirmed findings indicating that somatic symptoms are reliably correlated with history of menstrual difficulty.

These studies suggest that the nine months of pregnancy are filled with changing emotions. The majority of women report increases in anxiety, depression, crying, and lability of mood. Anxiety is lowest in the second and highest in the third trimesters; but there are no significant trimester differences noted for depression. The lability of mood reported by many women may account for the lack of consistent and strong findings regarding emotions in pregnancy.

## ANXIETY IN PREGNANCY AS A PREDICTOR OF DIFFICULTIES IN DELIVERY

Grimm (1967) studied the relationship of "psychological tension" as measured by the TAT to certain objective aspects of the course of pregnancy: weight gain, length of labor, complications during labor and delivery, and physical status of the child. Using a sample of 200 women, she found that both the amount of weight gained and the length of the second stage of labor were significantly related to the tension index. The tension index was not significantly related to total length of labor, complications, or physical status of the infant. Davids, DeVault, and Talmadge (1961) had found that a significantly greater proportion of women who had normal deliveries perceived a pregnant woman on card 2 of the TAT and drew a female figure on the Draw-a-Person. Grimm predicted that those women who (1) did not perceive the woman on card 2 as pregnant (NP), (2) drew a male figure first (M), and (3) obtained a high tension index would be more likely to have a complication of pregnancy or childbirth. Neither the NP or the M score significantly correlated with any of the four outcome criteria. However, of the 200 women, 11 obtained a high tension index, an NP score, and an M score. Twenty-seven percent of these 11 women had an infant who died or was deformed whereas only 3% of the remainder of the sample had such a child, a highly significant finding.

Davids, DeVault, and Talmadge (1961) used the Manifest Anxiety Scale (a 50-item true-false inventory referring to physical and emotional feelings commonly believed to be indicative of anxiety), in addition to the Wechsler intelligence test, the Thematic Apperception Test, the Sentence Completion Test, and Maternal Personality Ratings (7-point ratings on 12 scales). Forty-eight women were evaluated in the seventh month of pregnancy and again postdelivery. All tests were scored independently. The delivery room record of each woman was then evaluated and categorized as normal or abnormal on the basis of any problems with delivery and/or with the health of the infant. The results indicated a significantly greater amount of anxiety reported in the seventh month of pregnancy by women who later fell into the abnormal group than by those experiencing normal deliveries.

Although anxiety scores for both groups decreased postpartum, group differences were maintained.

In a second sample of 50 patients, Davids and DeVault (1962), using a similar methodology, again obtained higher anxiety scores on the Manifest Anxiety Scale for the abnormal delivery group. Differences were also found on the TAT cards scored for anxiety, the rating of maternal anxiety (by the psychologists), self-rating scales of anxiety, and the Sentence Completion Test. Davids and DeVault concluded that mothers who later had difficulty in the delivery room showed markedly more anxiety in the third trimester than did those having normal deliveries.

McDonald and Christakos (1963), also evaluating women in the third trimester (seventh month), found significantly higher scores on the Manifest Anxiety Scale and on a majority of scales on the Minnesota Multiphasic Personality Inventory (the MMPI, a statistically derived questionnaire consisting of 565 questions in a true-false format) for women who fell into the abnormal delivery group. The distinction of abnormal versus normal delivery was made according to standard clinical criteria.

McDonald and Parham (1964), using the Manifest Anxiety Scale (MAS), the MMPI, and Kent Intelligence Scales, tested 160 unwed primigravidas in the third trimester. Consistent with findings concerning married women (McDonald & Christakos, 1963), higher mean scores for the abnormal delivery group were noted on the MAS and MMPI scales.

Zuckerman, Nurnberger, Gardiner, Vandiveer, Barrett, and den Breeijen (1963) tested 49 primiparous, lower to middle-class women during the fourth or fifth month of pregnancy. The MAS, AACL, Parental Attitude Research Instrument (PARI), MF Scale of MMPI, and a Somatic Complaint Inventory were used. The test scores were correlated with the length of labor and the amount of anesthesia administered. The results indicated that the length of labor was not related to the MAS, AACL (scored for anxiety), PARI, or M-F Scale. A significant correlation between the scores on the AACL and the amount of anesthesia administered was found.

A series of investigations concerning anxiety has attempted to study trait-state anxiety during pregnancy (Spielberger, 1966). The trait-state anxiety theory conceptualizes two different types of anxiety. *State anxiety* is the emotional reaction of an individual to a situation that is perceived as dangerous or threatening. The reaction may vary in intensity and duration. Furthermore, it may fluctuate over time as a function of the stress impinging upon the individual, the individual's perception of the stress, and/or the individual's adaptation to the stress. *Trait anxiety* is a person's anxiety proneness; that is, the tendency of an individual to perceive situations as threatening or dangerous. People high in trait anxiety are more likely to perceive danger or threat in situations than are people low in trait anxiety. Spielberger, Gorsuch, and Lushene (1970) developed the State-Trait Anxiety Inventory (STAI), based on the trait-state model, for the evaluation of emotional reactions to stress. The STAI consists of two scales: the A-State Scale and the A-Trait Scale. The A-State Scale consists of 20 statements reflecting levels of anxiety at a particular moment. The A-Trait Scale consists of 20 items concerning how one generally feels.

Edwards and Jones (1970) administered the STAI A-Trait and A-State Scales at the beginning of the third trimester to 53 unwed pregnant women. The STAI A-State was also given each week until delivery. The women classified as having normal deliveries showed a reduction in state anxiety six weeks prior to delivery. This lowered A-State was relatively consistent until one week prior to delivery, at which time there was a significant increase in A-State. Women who later had complications demonstrated a different pattern of response in that they remained at a consistently high A-State until one week before delivery, at which time their A-State level dramatically decreased.

Gorsuch and Key (1974) used the STAI A-Trait and A-State Scales with 118 low-income women at the first visit to the obstetrician; they readministered the A-State at each subsequent visit. After delivery the women were classified as normal or abnormal either on the basis of obstetric complications during the third trimester or delivery or on the basis of abnormalities of the neonate. There were no differences between the two groups on trait anxiety; however, the groups differed with regard to A-State. Women with obstetric complications reported significantly higher levels of A-State during the third and fourth lunar months (first trimester). There were no significant differences during the ninth and tenth lunar months, although the abnormal group scored higher in A-State. Gorsuch and Key concluded that anxiety during the first months of pregnancy is dysfunctional.

The apparent discrepancy between the Gorsuch and Key study and previous studies using the Manifest Anxiety Scale or projective tests to measure anxiety may be explained by the instruments used. It appears reasonable to assume that the MAS and STAI are in fact tapping different aspects of anxiety. The MAS could be significantly affected by life changes or other external events, whereas the STAI may be tapping a more internal or perhaps physiologic type of anxiety. If this is the case, one could hypothesize that anxiety as measured by the STAI is more dysfunctional in the first trimester, whereas anxiety as measured by the MAS is more dysfunctional in the third trimester. One could predict that high scores on the STAI during the first trimester would be correlated with congenital abnormalities or other problems in the neonate not directly related to the process of delivery. Those women who had high states of anxiety during the third trimester as measured by the MAS would be more likely to deliver prematurely or to have longer or more difficult labors; however, problems with the infant would be the result of either prematurity or the process of delivery.

The majority of studies have found significant differences in anxiety between women who experience difficulty in labor and delivery and those women who do not (Davids, DeVault, & Talmadge, 1961; McDonald & Christakos, 1963; McDonald & Parham, 1964). The studies that used the MAS were methodologically sound and revealed no differences in anxiety during pregnancy with regard to age, intelligence, or parity. The majority of studies finding problems of labor and delivery correlated with anxiety noted anxiety differences in the third trimester. Zuckerman et al. (1963) failed to find a relationship between anxiety and problems in delivery; however, they tested women in the second trimester and this may account for their lack of findings. This hypothesis gains some support from Zemlick and Watson (1953), who found that anxiety measures became more significantly correlated with difficulties in labor and delivery as the pregnancy progressed; that is, measures of anxiety in the third trimester were more significantly correlated to difficulties in labor and delivery than were the findings of the same instruments in the second trimester.

A major criticism of all studies of anxiety during pregnancy as a predictor of difficulties in labor and delivery is the outcome criteria. The definition of difficulty in labor or obstetric complications varies from study to study. A variety of outcome criteria have been used: total length of labor, length of second stage of labor, difficulties in labor, or problems in the pregnancy. Some of these criteria are quite subjective and often the same obstetrician provided the predictive ratings as well as determined the outcome ratings. Finally, none of the studies dealing with problems in the neonate provided data from neonatologists; rather, subjective or broad diagnostic categories were used and the infants were evaluated by the obstetrician.

There does appear to be a significant negative relationship between high anxiety and several assessments utilizing the MAS and the STAI over all three trimesters in a large sample. The effects of such variables as age, race, SES, marital status, parity, and gravidity must be controlled before any definite conclusions regarding the role of anxiety in pregnancy can be reached.

## DEGREE OF PSYCHOPATHOLOGY

A series of studies has used the MMPI to evaluate the emotional stability of women during pregnancy. This test is comprised of 3 validity scales and 10 clinical scales. The scores on each scale are plotted on a profile sheet, which can then be interpreted by using either actuarial or clinical methods or a combination of both. Hooke and Marks (1962) compared the profiles of 24 women in the eighth month of pregnancy with those of a normative female sample. The 3 validity scales, 10 clinical scales, and 4 new scales—ego strength, responsibility, dependency, and low back pain—were used. Differences were found on 10 of the 17 scales, but testing for percentage differences of abnormal scores did not yield a reliable split. T scores of 70 or above were found in approximately 15% of the profiles of each group. The authors noted the absence of mild subjective discomfort, such as anxiety or depression, as well as the low incidence of psychopathology of any kind. In reviewing their findings, they concluded that pregnancy is a period of good psychological adjustment and emotional health.

Osborne (1977a) hypothesized that more salient differences between pregnant and nonpregnant women might be noted in the first trimester of pregnancy. The Minnesota Multiphasic Personality Inventory scores of 94 pregnant women were compared to those of female medical patients. The 10 clinical scales, 3 validity scales, and 4 research scales (tired housewife, ego strength, anxiety, and repression) were used. The medical patient group obtained significantly higher scores on all clinical scales except paranoid (Pa) and social introversion (Si). Among the three validity scales, F was significantly elevated in the medical patients. There were differences on the four research scales as well, with the medical group higher on tired housewife (TH) and factor A (anxiety), whereas the pregnant group was higher on ego strength (Es).

In a later study, Osborne (1978) investigated changes between the first and the third trimester on the MMPI by retesting his initial sample. He noted significant decreases on the F Scale (a validity scale on which high scores reflect a tendency to put one's self in a bad light). Ratings on depression (D), masculinity-femininity (M-F), tired housewife (Th), and anxiety were also significantly lower. The decrease reflected a decrease in distress, along with fewer concerns about the problems of managing a house and family. The lower M-F probably reflected a shift in interest patterns in the feminine direction as the pregnancy progressed. It appears that women become more comfortable as the pregnancy progresses.

One could interpret these results as suggesting that pregnancy is a time of emotional and psychological changes. The first trimester appears to be one in which depression and anxiety are relatively pronounced and women are concerned over home and family. The third trimester seems to show a decrease in subjective distress and concern over house and family.

Osborne (1977b) also used the MMPI to study the effects of previous pregnancies on a woman's psychological adjustment during pregnancy. Ninety-four women in the third trimester of pregnancy were administered the Minnesota Multiphasic Personality Inventory. The scores of 52 multigravidas and 42 primigravidas were compared. There were no differences on either the validity scales or the research scales: tired housewife, ego strength, factor A (anxiety), and factor R (repression). On the clinical scales two significant differences were noted: on hysteria multigravidas scored significantly higher but on hypomania they scored significantly lower. The author noted that the differences on the latter scale might be the result of age since scores on this scale decline with age and the multigravida group was older. It appears that multigravidas may adopt repression and denial as defense mechanisms more often and that they may have less energy than primigravidas. Overall, the subjective and emotional response to pregnancy as measured by the MMPI appears similar for multigravidas and primigravidas.

Studies using the Minnesota Multiphasic Personality Inventory suggest that pregnancy is a period of relatively little emotional distress. There are indications, however, of a shift in interests over the course of the pregnancy, as well as of a relative decrease in anxiety and depression. Multigravidas appear to have less energy and to adopt repression and denial as defense mechanisms more frequently than do primigravidas.

## PHYSICAL SYMPTOMS

### Sick Role Expectations

Illness involves social as well as biological factors in that a person who is ill may be excused from normal duties and functions. Thus, being sick may cause a change in roles or even a change in status. For the hypochondriac, the person who is not physically sick but functions or behaves as though he or she were, illness may be a solution to difficulties in fulfilling traditional roles. Illness legitimizes a person's inability to fulfill those roles and provides a new role for him or her. Thus, a person's motivation to assume a sick role could have social origins.

Pregnancy is a normal process involving biological changes; thus, one would expect that social factors may be involved in the motivation to assume a sick role. Rosengren (1961) hypothesized that factors such as social status, social aspirations, and social mobility might be correlated with the assumption of a sick role by a pregnant woman.

The sick role is defined in this body of research as based on (1) exemption from normal responsibilities during pregnancy, (2) pregnancy viewed as a "condition" that one has to "get over," (3) extent of concern and anxiety about organicity and body changes during pregnancy, (4) acceptance of pain and suffering as natural corollaries of one's being "ill" and getting "well," and (5) extent of acceptance of a subordinate role vis-à-vis the doctor (Davids & Rosengren, 1962; Rosengren, 1961).

Rosengren (1961) studied a group of pregnant women in which 44 were of lower socioeconomic status and 32 were of higher socioeconomic status. Sick role was negatively correlated with social aspirations and was positively related to material aspirations, lower socioeconomic status, and social mobility. Of some interest was the deviation of the occupational level of the woman from an otherwise consistent social class pattern. Women who had been or were employed in higher status occupations tended to regard themselves as more sick than did those who had held lower status positions. It was hypothesized that for the higher occupation women, pregnancy involved a drop in status whereas for the lower status women it involved an increase in status.

Davids and Rosengren (1962) evaluated the psychological status of those women assuming a sick role as opposed to those who did not. The factor of social stability was also examined. Thirty women who were of high socioeconomic status were seen during the second trimester of pregnancy. The women were assessed in terms of sick role expectations, social dissatisfaction, conflicts in basic cultural values (pertaining to social class), self-esteem on the basis of self-ratings with respect to five social attributes, and an objective index of socioeconomic status. The psychological measures included the Wechsler intelligence test, the Manifest Anxiety Scale, and selected Thematic Apperception Test cards. The TAT stories were scored in terms of alienation. The women were also asked to provide a happiness self-rating and to rate their happiness about being pregnant. Finally, each woman was rated during the interview on 12 personality characteristics. The total rating resulted in either a negative or a positive personality picture.

Social instability was positively associated with scores on the MAS. The more socially dissatisfied the woman, the higher her manifest anxiety. These women also tended to be less happy that they were pregnant. Women who expressed conflicts with cultural values were also less happy to be pregnant.

Significant differences in emotional adjustment were found between high and low socioeconomic groups. Higher socioeconomic status women also reported significantly higher scores on the degree of happiness they believed would be attributed to them by other people. Additionally, these women obtained more positive ratings from the examining psychologist. This might have been a reflection of their adjustment or of a similarity in values between these women and the examiners.

These findings are consistent with the idea that certain women perceive pregnancy as a period of illness rather than a normal condition. This type of role expectation would be more likely to occur if a woman had low socioeconomic status, were experiencing social mobility, or had values that conflicted with cultural values. For such women, pregnancy tends to be viewed as an illness and they are likely to experience anxiety and unhappiness. Thus, a woman's adjustment during pregnancy may depend upon the social function a sick role can serve.

## Nausea and Vomiting

Psychological factors have long been suspected of playing a role in the nausea and vomiting experienced by some women during pregnancy. One of the most frequently cited studies was conducted by Robertson (1946).

He hypothesized that nausea and vomiting are an expression of disgust and postulated three factors as characteristic of women with this reaction: frigidity or aversion to sex, undue attachment to mother, and a history of dyspepsia. He interviewed 100 married pregnant women and classified them according to severity of symptoms. Of the sample, almost half (43) had no symptoms, 31 had minor symptoms, 17 had moderate symptoms, and 9 had severe symptoms. The interview data revealed significant differences among the four groups with regard to frequency of intercourse (with the highest frequency reported by the symptom-free group). A similar trend was found with differences in overattachment to mother.

Rosen (1955) studied women during the first trimester to determine whether stress is a significant factor in nausea and vomiting. Using an interview technique, he concluded that the severity of symptoms was caused by emotional stress experienced by the women during pregnancy.

Coppen (1958), using a psychiatric interview and personality questionnaire, studied 50 randomly selected primiparas. Twenty-nine had some vomiting and 21 were symptom-free. He found no differences between the women who experienced vomiting and those who did not in extroversion, neurotic symptoms, sexual functioning, stress, or attitudes toward pregnancy.

Rejection of the pregnancy as a factor in nausea was suggested in psychoanalytic theory (Deutsch, 1945) but has not found support in the literature. A sample of 212 women was studied by Poffenberger, Poffenberger, and Landis (1952). A total of 55% reported nausea, but there was no relationship between intent to become pregnant and nausea. Similar results were reported by Nilsson, Kaij, and Jacobson (1967).

Chertok, Mondzain, and Bonnaud (1963) suggested that ambivalence toward the child, not simple rejection, is the crucial variable in excessive vomiting. They followed 100 primiparous women from the third month of pregnancy to childbirth. Data were obtained through semistructured interviews. Women were classified as vomiting only if emesis of stomach content occurred. Ordinary nausea was not considered. Sixty-seven percent of the subjects vomited during pregnancy. Mild vomiting occurred in 53 of the 67 vomiters and severe vomiting occurred in 14 (29%). Attitude toward the child was rated in three categories: wanting, rejecting, and ambivalent. The research unit (which had carried out both classifications) found a statistically significant positive relationship between vomiting and ambivalence toward the child. Cognizant of the potential influence of experimenter bias, Chertok et al. asked different judges independently to classify the 100 cases with regard to attitude toward the child. These results showed the same trend but were not statistically significant.

Uddenberg, Nilsson, and Almgren (1971) studied 152 women during the second trimester, immediately after parturition, and six months postpartum. The women were placed into one of three categories as follows: no nausea (31%), slight to moderate nausea (47%), and pronounced nausea (22%). A questionnaire, a self-rating scale, and two projective tests were used. The authors found that the presence and degree of nausea were not associated with age, parity, or marital status. Both the "no nausea" and "pronounced nausea" groups acknowledged a greater number of symptoms on the Neurosis Scale (a 32-item questionnaire) and had more mental disturbance postpartum than the "moderate nausea" group. The "pronounced nausea" group also had more emotional difficulties during pregnancy. The authors concluded that the "moderate nausea" group was the healthiest psychologically. They noted that consistent with psychoanalytic theory, this group also reported a stronger identification with their mothers. The "no nausea" group, much like the "perfect pregnancy" described by Deutsch (1945), were more identified with their fathers. Although having no problems with the pregnancy, they had difficulties postpartum.

Netter-Munkut, Marc, and Konig (1972), using Eysenck's scales, found no relationship between degree of neuroticism and nausea and vomiting in pregnancy.

Palmer (1973) studied 138 white primigravidas during the first 12–16 weeks of pregnancy and 4 weeks later. Sixty-six reported vomiting (48%). Vomiters were compared with nonvomiters on five measures: interview, physical indices of obesity and body shape, psychoneurotic symptom status (the Middlesex Hospital Questionnaire), the Eysenck Personality Inventory, and the Semantic Differential. He found a significant excess of vomiters in social classes 4 and 5 and a deficit in social classes 1 and 2 (the husband's or woman's father's occupation was used to determine class). No differences were noted with regard to marital or educational status, personal and family history of psychiatric treatment, age at menarche, smoking, or history of operative surgery. A physical difference was noted between the two groups: the vomiters were shorter. No differences were noted in anxiety, phobic anxiety, obsessionality, depression, or hysteria as measured by the Middlesex Hospital Questionnaire. Significant differences were noted on the Somatic Symptom Scale, with vomiters reporting more symptoms. The Eysenck Personality Inventory did not differentiate between the two groups on either introversion-extroversion or neuroticism. The findings on the Semantic Differential were largely negative and were attributed to chance. The findings of this study were largely negative, supporting the notion that nausea and vomiting in pregnancy cannot be viewed as indicators of emotional or psychological maladjustment.

Although theoretically sound, the idea that nausea and vomiting during pregnancy may be related to psychological difficulties, such as ambivalent feelings regarding the child, has not found empirical support. It appears that vomiting during pregnancy occurs frequently (50–70% of women) and is generally unrelated either to emotional factors such as neuroticism or to negative or ambivalent feelings toward the child.

The syndrome of hyperemesis of pregnancy (hyperemesis gravidarum) whereby vomiting, usually in the first or second trimester, becomes so severe that the mother's life and pregnancy are jeopardized, can result in medical hospitalization. This condition can be accompanied by significant weight loss, malnutrition (particularly important in this sensitive period of fetal development), and volume depletion. Hospitalization may be necessary to sustain adequate fluid and nutritional intake via intravenous routes. In clinical practice psychological mechanisms have been thought to contribute to this rather severe and occasionally life-threatening problem. Clinical impression suggests that these women seem to be relatively young, emotionally unsupported, prima-gravidas in conflict with an important person or persons about the pregnancy. The treatment of hospitalization, intravenous fluids, sedation, and isolation from stressful environmental circumstances, particularly family and domestic pressures, usually rapidly results in decrease of vomiting and restoration of adequate oral intake. Discharge of the patient to the same environment, unmodified from what it was during the development of the original symptoms, may result in the return of the disorder. Environmental manipulation and conjoint family therapy seem more useful than individual psychodynamically oriented psychotherapy in such cases. Improvement with these techniques suggests that psychological mechanisms may contribute to the nausea and vomiting. However, there are well documented physiological changes which occur in pregnancy which produce a diathesis for nausea and vomiting. Such changes include a decrease in the rate of gastric emptying, a decrease in peristalsis, and an increase in gut transit time. Exogenously administered estrogen, in nonpregnant women, frequently produces nausea and even vomiting as a side effect. The increased levels of estrogen and placental gonadotropins in pregnancy may provide a physiological basis for morning sickness as well as for more severe forms of vomiting.

## Cravings and Aversions

Cravings, or compulsive desires, for certain foods is believed to be so frequent in normal pregnant women that this phenomenon is often a target of humor. Aversions, or the distaste for certain foods or drinks eaten before pregnancy, have also been noted. A more atypical phenomenon, the craving for a substance normally regarded as inedible, may occur in certain pregnant women.

Most studies have indicated that one-third to two-thirds of women (regardless of race or geographic region) experience cravings and/or aversions at some time during the pregnancy. Posner, McCottrey, and Posner (1957) found cravings in 66% of 600 women; Taggart (1961), in a study of primigravidas, found two-thirds developed cravings, usually for fruit, and that aversions were as common as cravings. Dickens and Trethowan (1971), in a study of 100 women, found 51 primigravidas with cravings and 62 with aversions.

The range of foods or drinks to which an aversion or a craving has been reported is quite large; however, Dickens and Trethowan (1971) noted that certain patterns emerge, with sweet, sour, savory, or salty substances being frequently cited. Fruit (fizzy fruit drinks included) is the most popularly craved item. Two other groups—sweet items such as jelly or ice cream and vegetables, including nuts and pickles—are equally common and are the next most craved items. Additionally, there is some suggestion that texture as well as taste is important (Posner et al., 1957); that is, the woman enjoys biting or chewing something hard or crisp (for example, apples are preferred to oranges).

Aversions are less well documented; however, tea and coffee were noted in several studies (Dickens & Trethowan, 1971; Taggart, 1961). Cravings for these substances are rare and Dickens and Trethowan's findings suggest that cravings and aversions are for the most part antithetical and may have an inverse relationship with each other.

Several psychological theories have been advanced to account for these changes in appetite. Deutsch (1945) suggested that food cravings express a conflict regarding the fetus. She theorized that the compulsive eating of food, which commonly represents fecundation, may represent an "obsessive undoing" of an unconscious wish to destroy the child; however, the research literature has failed to support this idea.

Dickens and Trethowan (1971) evaluated 100 primigravidas after delivery and found no correlation between appetite disorders and factors that might suggest a rejection of the pregnancy. The factors examined in their study included such issues as whether the pregnancy was planned, the attitude of the husband, the financial impact of the pregnancy, and anxiety related to childbirth. None of these was correlated with appetite disorders. They did find that the number of women who smoked, took alcohol, or had had a previous change in appetite under emotional stress was significantly higher in any of the three appetite categories (cravings, aversions, or both). In any event, the incidence of appetite disturbance during pregnancy is quite high and does not appear to be related to maternal rejection, difficulties in pregnancy and labor, or prematurity. Thus, a healthy pregnancy, both psychologically and physically, may be characterized by an appetite disturbance and there appear to be no serious consequences to mother or infant. Dickens and Trethowan interpreted these findings to suggest that there is some predisposition to oral fixation in those women who develop appetite disorders. Factors such as suggestion, imitation, identification, and attention seeking may be the psychological mechanisms responsible.

Another factor that Dickens & Trethowan (1971) deemed worthy of more attention with regard to appetite change during pregnancy was alteration in taste. They cited two studies that documented alterations in taste: Hansen and Langer in 1935, using dilute solutions, and Caresano and Minazzi in 1965, using a more precise electrical method, found that the threshold for taste is considerably higher and more variable during pregnancy. If these findings are representative, then the preference of pregnant women for sweet, spicy, salty, or sour substances is understandable, as is dislike of bland or delicate foods. Furthermore, the choice of substances such as apples, which must be bitten and chewed, may in some way compensate for decreased taste.

Henkin (1971) reviews taste abnormalities (decreased taste sensitivity and perverted taste) in pregnant women (and other patients) particularly in the first trimester of pregnancy. He describes abnormalities of zinc metabolism, particularly zinc deficiencies, which he feels are responsible for the taste abnormalities.

Although change in taste threshold may contribute to variations in food preferences during pregnancy, this factor alone would certainly not account for compulsive preferences or aversions. Rather, an interaction of psychological and physiological factors must be at work.

## PSYCHOLOGICAL ASPECTS OF PREGNANCY: CONCEPTUALIZING OUTCOME

The studies reviewed in this chapter suggest a conceptual framework within which one can view a woman's psychological reaction to a pregnancy. It appears that two very important factors affecting the initial acceptance of a pregnancy are number of previous children and space between previous pregnancies. Initial acceptance of a pregnancy is not universal; in fact, approximately 50% of the time a woman's reaction to the news of pregnancy will be rejection or ambivalence. Initial rejection or ambivalence will probably dissipate as the pregnancy progresses, and by the third trimester most women have positive feelings about the pregnancy.

The emotionality of pregnant women is frequently noted in popular writings and is supported by research findings. The vast majority of women experience mood changes, increased emotional responsiveness, and depression. Symptoms of fatigue, irritability, insomnia, and weeping are commonly noted; however, these emotional changes are not so severe as to be reflected in deviant or pathological scores on objective tests of psychopathology.

Changes in anxiety during pregnancy have been the subject of many research studies. Few have dealt with fluctuations in anxiety during the course of a normal pregnancy; however, those that have addressed this question have suggested that anxiety is lowest during the second trimester.

High levels of anxiety during the third trimester, as measured by the

Thematic Apperception Test and the Manifest Anxiety Scale, are positively correlated with somatic complaints, difficult deliveries, and/or problems with the infant. Studies that used the State-Trait Anxiety Inventory found that high levels of anxiety during the first trimester are dysfunctional and are positively correlated with obstetric complications. A possible explanation for these seemingly contradictory findings is that the instruments tap two different types of anxiety. Each may be correlated with specific difficulties in labor, delivery, or the health of the neonate; however, the generality of the outcome criterion utilized thus far does not allow this type of distinction to be made.

Body image changes are not well documented by research. Although such changes are frequently mentioned in clinical studies, the few research studies have yielded contradictory results. In view of the physical changes in a woman's body during pregnancy, it appears logical to hypothesize that corresponding psychological changes also take place. Perhaps the use of more sophisticated and sensitive criterion measures will yield more clear-cut results.

Sexual interest and sexual behavior also appear to be affected by pregnancy, although the mechanisms underlying the changes are unclear. The majority of women report a significant decrease in both sexual interest and frequency of intercourse during the third trimester of pregnancy. This decrease is only transient, however, and most women report a return to prepregnancy frequency of coitus.

Physical symptoms appear to be present in the average pregnancy. Although nausea and vomiting have been thought to be related to psychological difficulties such as ambivalence toward the fetus, it appears that this is not the case. Moderate vomiting occurs frequently during pregnancy and is unrelated to emotional factors. Changes in appetite also occur frequently, with one-third to two-thirds of women experiencing cravings and/or aversions at some time during the pregnancy. These changes in appetite are not related to attitudes toward the fetus, difficulties in delivery, or health of the fetus. One hypothesis is that appetite disturbances occur in women in whom there is a predisposition to oral fixation. Another potential explanation is based on changes in taste thresholds during pregnancy. The most reasonable theory suggests that extreme changes in appetite such as cravings or aversions are probably the result of an interaction of psychological and physiological factors.

Interpersonal relationships may affect the course of a pregnancy. The literature to date suggests that a woman's relationship with her own mother may affect her psychologically during a pregnancy. It is assumed that a woman's feminine identification and comfort with regard to her impending maternal role have their origin in her relationship with her own mother. A woman who feels comfortable in accepting the responsibilities and role changes implied by motherhood is assumed to experience less psychological distress and conflict during pregnancy.

A woman's relationship with her husband appears to be a major factor in determining how well she is able to cope with the numerous physical and emotional changes brought about by pregnancy. It is important for both partners to recognize that emotional lability, nausea and vomiting, appetite disturbances, and decreased sexual interest are all typical of a normal pregnancy. Perhaps of equal importance, both partners may need the reassurance that these changes are transient and can best be dealt with by open communication and mutual understanding and support.

## REFERENCES

BIBRING, L. Some considerations of the psychological processes in pregnancy. *Psychoanalytic Study of the Child,* 1959, *14,* 113-121.

BIBRING, L., DWYER, F., HUNTINGTON, S., and VALENSTEIN, A. A study of the psychological processes in pregnancy and of the earliest mother-child relationship. Part 1: Some propositions and comments. *Psychoanalytic Study of the Child,* 1961, *16,* 9-24. (a)

———. A study of the psychological processes in pregnancy and of the earliest mother-child relationship. Part 2: Methodological considerations. *Psychoanalytic Study of the Child,* 1961, *16,* 25-72. (b)

BIBRING, L., and VALENSTEIN, A. Psychological aspects of pregnancy. *Clinical Obstetrics and Gynecology,* 1976, *19,* 357-371.

BIELE, M. Unwanted pregnancy: symptom of depressive practice. *American Journal of Psychiatry,* 1971, *128,* 104-110.

BLOS, P. *On adolescence.* New York: Free Press, 1962.

BUSHNELL, L. F. First trimester depression: a suggested treatment. *Obstetrics and Gynecology,* 1961, *18,* 281-282.

CAPLAN, G. Psychological aspects of maternity care. *American Journal of Public Health,* 1957, *47,* 25-31.

CARESANO, G., and MINAZZI, M. Taste sensitivity in pregnancy and puerperium. Cited in W. H. Trethowan and G. Dickens, Cravings, aversions, and pica of pregnancy. In John G. Howells (ed.), *Modern perspectives in psycho-obstetrics.* New York: Bruner/Mazel, 1972.

CHERTOK, L., MONDZAIN, M. L., and BONNAUD, M. Vomiting and the wish to have a child. *Psychosomatic Medicine,* 1963, *25,* 13-17.

COLEMAN, D. Psychological state during first pregnancy, *American Journal of Orthopsychiatry,* 1969, *39,* 788-797.

COLEMAN, D., and COLMAN, L. *Pregnancy: the psychological experience.* New York: Seabury, 1971.

COPPEN, A. J. Psychosomatic aspects of pre-eclamptic toxemia. *Journal of Psychosomatic Research,* 1958, *2,* 241-265.

DALTON, K. Prospective study. *British Journal of Psychiatry,* 1971, *118,* 689-692.

DAVIDS, A., and DEVAULT, S. Use of the TAT and human figure drawings in research on personality, pregnancy, and perception. *Journal of Projective Techniques,* 1960, *24,* 362-365.

———. Maternal anxiety during pregnancy and childbirth abnormalities. *Psychosomatic Medicine,* 1962, *24,* 464-470.

DAVIDS, A., DEVAULT, S., and TALMADGE, M. Psychological study of emotional factors in pregnancy: a preliminary report. *Psychosomatic Medicine,* 1961, *23,* 93–103.

DAVIDS, A., and HOLDEN, R. H. Consistency of maternal attitudes and personality from pregnancy to eight months following childbirth. *Developmental Psychology,* 1970, *2,* 364–366.

DAVIDS, A., and ROSENGREN, R. Social stability and psychological adjustment during pregnancy. *Psychosomatic Medicine,* 1962, *24,* 579–583.

DESPRES, M. A. Favorable and unfavorable attitudes toward pregnancy in primiparae. *Journal of Genetic Psychology,* 1937, *51,* 241.

DEUTSCH, H. *The psychology of women.* Vol. 1: *Motherhood.* New York: Grune & Stratton, 1945.

DICKENS, G., and TRETHOWAN, W. H. Cravings and aversions during pregnancy. *Journal of Psychosomatic Research,* 1971, *15,* 259–268.

EDWARDS, C. H., MCDONALD, S., MITCHELL, J. R., JONES, L., MASON, L., and TRIGG, D. Effect of clay and cornstarch intake on women and their infants. *Journal of the American Dietetic Association,* 1965, *41,* 109–115.

EDWARDS, C. H., MCSWAIN, S., and HAIRE, S. Odd dietary practices of women. *Journal of the American Dietetic Association,* 1954, *30,* 976–978.

EDWARDS, K. R., and JONES, M. R. Personality changes related to pregnancy and obstetric complications. *Proceedings of the 78th Annual Convention of the American Psychological Association,* 1970, Vol. 5 341–342.

ERIKSON, E. G. *Childhood and society.* (2nd ed.) New York: Norton, 1963.

FALICOV, C. J. Sexual adjustment during first pregnancy and post partum. *American Journal of Obstetrics and Gynecology,* 1971, *117,* 991–1000.

FISHER, S., and CLEVELAND, S. E. *Body image and personality.* Princeton: Van Nostrand, 1958.

FISHER, S., and RECHTER, J. Selective effects of the menstrual experience upon aniseikonic body perception. *Psychosomatic Medicine,* 1970, Vol *31* 365–371.

FLOYD, J., and VINEY, L. Ego identity and ego ideal in the unwed mother. *British Journal of Medical Psychology,* 1974, *47,* 273–281.

GOODLIN, R. C., KELLER, D. W., and RAFFIN, M. Orgasm during late pregnancy: possible deleterious effects. *Obstetrics and Gynecology,* 1971, *38,* 916–920.

GORDON, E. M. Acceptance of pregnancy before and since oral contraception. *Obstetrics and Gynecology,* 1967, *29,* 144–146.

GORDON, E. M., KAPOSTINS, E. and GORDON, K. Factors in postpartum emotional adjustment. *American Journal of Orthopsychiatry,* 1965, *37,* 359–360.

GORSUCH, R. L., and KEY, K. Abnormalities of pregnancy as a function of anxiety and life stress. *Psychosomatic Medicine,* 1974, *36,* 352–362.

GRIFFITH, S. Pregnancy as an event with crisis potential for marital partners: a study of interpersonal needs. *Journal of Obstetric, Gynecologic, and Neonatal Nursing,* 1976, *5* 35–38.

GRIMM, R. Psychological tension in pregnancy. *Psychosomatic Medicine,* 1961, *23,* 520–526.

———. Psychological and social factors in pregnancy, delivery, and outcome. In S. A. Richardson and A. F. Guttmacher (eds.), *Childbearing: its social and psychological aspects.* Baltimore: Williams and Wilkins, 1967.

GRUDZINSKAS, J. C., WATSON, C., CHARD, T. Does Sexual Intercourse Cause Fetal Distress? *Lancet,* 1979, *2,* 692–693.

HANSEN R. and LANGER W. Changes of taste in pregnancy. Cited in John G. Howells (ed.), *Modern perspectives in psycho-obstetrics.* New York: Bruner/Mazel, 1972.

HEIMAN, M. Psychiatric complications: a psychoanalytic view of pregnancy. In J. J. Rowinsky and A. F. Guttmacher (eds.), *Medical, surgical, and gynecologic complications of pregnancy.* Baltimore: Williams and Wilkins, 1964.

HENKIN, R. I., SCHECHTER, P. J., HOYE R., and MATTERN, C. F. T. Idiopathic hypogeusia with dysgeusia, hyposmia, and dysosmia: A new syndrome. *Journal of American Medical Association,* 1971, *217,* 434–440.

HOLLENDER, H., and MCGEHEE. J. B. The wish to be held during pregnancy. *Journal of Psychosomatic Research,* 1974, *18,* 193–197.

HOOKE, F., and MARKS, A. MMPI characteristics of pregnancy. *Journal of Clinical Psychology,* 1962, *18,* 316–317.

HOWELLS, JOHN G. (ED.), *Modern perspectives in psycho-obstetrics.* New York: Bruner/Mazel, 1972.

HURST, J. C., and STROUSSE, T. The origin of emotional factors in normal pregnancy women. *American Journal of Medical Science,* 1938, *196,* 95–97.

JARRAHI-ZADEH, A., KANE, F. J., JR., VAN DE CASTLE, R. L., LACHENBRUCH, P. A., and EWING, J. A. Emotional and cognitive changes in pregnancy and early puerperium. *British Journal of Psychiatry,* 1969, *115,* 797–805.

KANE, F. J., JR., HARMAN, W. J., JR., KEELER, M. H., and EWING, J. A. Emotional and cognitive disturbance in the early puerperium. *British Journal of Psychiatry,* 1968, *114,* 99–102.

KENNY, J. A. Sexuality of pregnant and breast feeding women. *Archives of Sexual Behavior,* 1973, *2,* 215–229.

KLEIN, H. R., POTTER, H. W., and DYKE, R. B. *Anxiety in pregnancy and childbirth.* New York: Hoeber, 1950.

KLUSMAN, L. E. Reduction of pain in childbirth by the alleviation of anxiety during pregnancy. *Journal of Consulting and Clinical Psychology,* 1975, *43,* 162–165.

KYNDELY, K. The sexuality of women in pregnancy and postpartum. *Journal of Obstetric, Gynecologic, and Neonatal Nursing,* 1978, *7,* 28–32.

LABARRE, M. Pregnancy in married adolescents. *American Journal of Orthopsychiatry,* 1968, *38,* 47–55.

LANDIS, J. T., POFFENBERGER, T., and POFFENBERGER, S. The effects of first pregnancy upon the sexual adjustment of 212 couples. *American Sociological Review,* 1950, *15,* 766–772.

LEIFER, M. Psychological changes accompanying pregnancy and motherhood. *Genetic Psychology Monographs,* 1977, *95,* 55–96.

LIEBENBERG, B. Expectant fathers. *Child and Family,* 1969, *8,* 265–277.

LORR, M., DASTON, P., and SMITH, I. R. An analysis of mood states. *Educational and Psychological Measurement,* 1967, *27,* 89–96.

LUBIN, B., GARDENER, H., and ROTH, A. Mood and somatic symptoms during pregnancy. *Psychosomatic Medicine,* 1975, *37,* 136–146.

MANN, C., and CUNNINGHAM, G. Coital cautions in pregnancy. *Medical Aspects of Human Sexuality,* 1972, *6,* 14–26.

MASTERS, W. H., and JOHNSON, V. E. *Human sexual response.* Boston: Little, Brown, 1966.

MCCONNELL, O. L., and DASTON, P. G. Body image changes in pregnancy. *Journal of Projective Techniques,* 1961, *25,* 451–456.

MCDONALD, R. L. The role of emotional factors in obstetric complications: a review. *Psychosomatic Medicine,* 1968, *30,* 222–237.

MCDONALD, R. L., and CHRISTAKOS, A. C. Relationship of emotional factors during pregnancy to obstetric complications. *American Journal of Obstetrics and Gynecology,* 1963, *86,* 341.

McDONALD, R. L., and PARHAM, K. J. Relationship of emotional changes during pregnancy to obstetric complications in unmarried primigravidae. *American Journal of Obstetrics and Gynecology,* 1964, *90,* 195.

MEANS, R., GRIMWADE, J., and WOOD, C. A possible relationship between anxiety in pregnancy and puerperal depression. *Journal of Psychosomatic Research,* 1976, *20,* 605–610.

MEYEROWITZ, H. Satisfaction during pregnancy. *Journal of Marriage and the Family,* 1970, *32,* 38–42.

MOORE, D. S. The body image in pregnancy. *Journal of Nurse-Midwifery,* 1978, *12,* 17–27.

MORRIS, N. Attitude survey in pregnancy. *Journal of Psychosomatic Research,* 1963, *8,* 83–84.

———. The frequency of sexual intercourse during pregnancy. *Archives of Sexual Behavior,* 1975, *4,* 501–507.

NAEYE, R. L. Coitus and Associated Amniotic Fluid Infections. New England Journal of Medicine, 1979, *301,* 1198–1200.

NETTER, P. Psychosomatic complaints and patterns of reproductive history. *Journal of Psychosomatic Research,* 1977, *21,* 105–113.

NETTER-MUNKUT, P., MARC, G., and KONIG, B. The dimension of neuroticism as a modifying factor in the association between biological conditions and nausea in pregnancy. *Journal of Psychosomatic Research,* 1972, *16,* 395–404.

NEUBARDT, S. Coitus during pregnancy. *Medical Aspects of Human Sexuality,* 1973, *12,* 197–199.

NEWTON, N. *Maternal emotions: a psychosomatic medicine monograph.* New York: Hoeber, 1955.

———. Emotions of pregnancy. *Clinical Obstetrics and Gynecology,* 1963, *6,* 639–668.

NILSSON, A., KAIJ, L., and JACOBSON, L. Post-partum mental disorder in an unselected sample: the importance of the unplanned pregnancy. *Journal of Psychosomatic Research,* 1967, *10,* 341–347.

NOTT, F., FRANKLIN, M., ARMITAGE, C., and GELDER, M. G. Hormonal changes in mood in the puerperium. *British Journal of Psychiatry,* 1976, *128,* 379–383.

OSBORNE, D. Comparison of MMPI scores of pregnant women and female medical patients. *Journal of Clinical Psychiatry,* 1977, *33,* 448–450. (a)

———. MMPI characteristics of multigravidas and primigravidas in the third trimester of pregnancy. *Psychological Reports,* 1977, *40,* 81–82. (b)

———. MMPI changes between the first and third trimesters of pregnancy. *Journal of Clinical Psychiatry,* 1978, *34,* 92–94.

PALMER, R. L. A psychosomatic study of vomiting. *Journal of Psychosomatic Research,* 1973, *17,* 303–308.

PARKER, L. L. Coitus during pregnancy. *Journal of Nurse-Midwifery,* 1974, *19,* 4–7.

PINES, D. Pregnancy and motherhood: interaction between fantasy and reality. *British Journal of Medical Psychology,* 1972, *45,* 333–343.

POFFENBERGER, S., POFFENBERGER, T., and LANDIS, J. T. Intent toward conception and the pregnancy experience. *American Sociological Review,* 1952, *17,* 616–620.

POSNER, L. B., McCOTTREY, C. M., and POSNER, A. C. Pregnancy craving and pica. *Obstetrics and Gynecology,* 1957, *9,* 270–272.

PRESSER, H. B. Early motherhood: ignorance or bliss? *Family Planning Perspectives,* 1976, *6,* 8–14.

ROBERTSON, G. Composium on nausea and vomiting of pregnancy. *Lancet,* 1946, *2,* 336–338.

Roehner, J. Fatherhood: in pregnancy and birth. *Journal of Nurse-Midwifery,* 1976, *21,* 13–18.

Rosen, S. Emotional factors in nausea and vomiting of pregnancy. *Psychiatric Quarterly,* 1955, *29,* 621–633.

Rosengren, W. R. Social source of pregnancy as illness or normality. *Social Forces,* 1961, *39,* 260–267.

Rubin, R. Maternal tasks in pregnancy. *Maternal-Child Nursing Journal,* 1975, *4,* 143–153.

Sears, R. R., Maccoby, E. C., and Levin, H. *Patterns of child rearing role.* Evanston, Ill: Row, Peterson, 1957.

Shereshefsky, M., and Yarrow, J. (eds.), *Psychological aspects of a first pregnancy and early postnatal adaptation.* New York: Raven, 1973.

Sherman, J. A. *On the psychology of women: a survey of empirical studies.* Springfield: Charles C Thomas, 1971.

Slade, P. D. Awareness of body dimensions during pregnancy: an analogue study. *Psychological Medicine,* 1977, *7,* 245–252.

Slate, W. G. Coitus as a cause of abortion. *Medical Aspects of Human Sexuality,* 1970, *4,* 25–32.

Solberg, D. A., Butler, J., and Wagner, N. N. Sexual behavior in pregnancy. *New England Journal of Medicine,* 1973, *228,* 1098–1103.

Spielberger, C. D., Gorsuch, R. L., and Lushene, R. E. *Manual for the state-trait anxiety inventory.* Palo Alto: Consulting Psychologists Press, 1970.

Spielberger, C. D., and Jacobs, G. A. Emotional reactions to the stress of pregnancy and obstetric complications. Paper presented to the fifth International Congress on Psychosomatic Obstetrics and Gynecology, Rome, 1977.

Swigar, M. E., Bowers, M. B., and Flick, S. Grieving and unplanned pregnancy. *Psychiatry,* 1976, *39,* 72–81.

Taggart, N. Food habits in pregnancy. *Proceedings of the Nutritional Society,* 1961, *20,* 35–38.

Tobin, S. M. Emotional depression during pregnancy. *Obstetrics and Gynecology,* 1957, *10,* 677.

Tod, E. D. M. Puerpural depression. *British Journal of Psychiatry,* 1971, *118,* 689–692.

Tolor, A., and DiGrazia, P. V. Sexual attitudes and behavior patterns during and following pregnancy. *Archives of Sexual Behavior,* 1976, *5,* 539–551.

———. The body image of pregnant women as reflected in their human figure drawings. *Journal of Clinical Psychology,* 1977, *33,* 566–571.

Tolor, A., Rice, F. J., and Lanctot, C. A. Personality patterns of couples practicing the temperature-rhythm method of birth control. *Journal of Sexual Research,* 1975, *11,* 119–133.

Trethowan, W. H. The couvade syndrome: some further observations. *Journal of Psychosomatic Research,* 1968, *12,* 107–115.

Uddenberg, N. Psychological aspects of sexual inadequacy in women. *Journal of Psychosomatic Research,* 1974, *18,* 33–47.

Uddenberg, N., and Hakanson, M. Aniseikonic body perception in pregnancy. *Journal of Psychosomatic Research,* 1972, *16,* 179–184.

Uddenberg, N., and Nilsson, L. The longitudinal course of para-natal emotional disturbance. *ACTA Psychiatrica Scandinavica,* 1975, *52,* 160–169.

Uddenberg, N., Nilsson, A., and Almgren, P. Nausea in pregnancy: psychological and psychosomatic aspects. *Journal of Psychosomatic Research,* 1971, *15,* 269–276.

Van de Castle, R. L., and Kinder, P. Dream content during pregnancy. *Psychophysiology,* 1968, *4,* 375.

VAN MUISWINKEL, J. Vulnerability expressed by a primigravida. *Maternal-Child Nursing Journal,* 1974, *3,* 219–237.

VINEY, L. L., AITKIN, M., and FLOYD, J. Self-regard and size of human figure drawings: an interactional analysis. *Journal of Clinical Psychology,* 1974, *30,* 581–586.

WAGNER, N. N., and SOLBERG, D. A. Pregnancy and sexuality. *Medical Aspects of Human Sexuality,* 1974, *8,* 44–79.

WALEKO, K. F. Manifestations of a multigravida's feelings of vulnerability. *Maternal-Child Nursing Journal,* 1974, *3,* 103–131.

WEINBERG, J. S. Body image disturbance in pregnancy: a review. *Journal of Obstetric, Gynecologic, and Neonatal Nursing,* 1978, *7,* 18–21.

WELLER, S. D. V. Pica. *Current Medicine and Drugs,* 1963, *3,* 1.

WENNER, N. D., COHEN, M. B., WEIGERT, E. V., KVARNES, R. G., OHANESON, E. M., and FEARING, J. M. Emotional problems in pregnancy. *Psychiatry,* 1969, *32,* 389–410.

WILLIAMS, C. C., WILLIAMS, R. A., GRISWOLD, M. J., and HOLMES, T. H. Pregnancy and life change. *Journal of Psychosomatic Research,* 1975, *19,* 123–129.

WINOKUR, K. G., and WERBOFF, J. The relationship of conscious maternal attitudes to certain aspects of pregnancy. *Psychiatry Quarterly Supplement,* 1956, *30,* 61–70.

WITTREICH, W. J., and RADCLIFFE, K. B. The influence of simulated mutilation upon the perception of the human figure. *Journal of Abnormal and Social Psychology,* 1955, *51,* 493–495.

WOLKIND, S. N. Psychological factors and the minor symptoms of pregnancy. *Journal of Psychosomatic Research,* 1974, *18,* 161–165.

———. Women who have been "in care": psychological and social status during pregnancy. *Journal of Child Psychology and Psychiatry,* 1977, *18,* 179–182.

ZEMLICK, M., and WATSON, R. Maternal attitudes of acceptance and rejection during and after pregnancy. *American Journal of Orthopsychiatry,* 1953, *23,* 570–575.

ZUCKERMAN, M., NURNBERGER, J. I., GARDINER, S. H., VANDIVEER, J. M., BARRETT, B. H., and DEN BREEIJEN, A. Psychological correlates of somatic complaints in pregnancy and difficulty in childbirth. *Journal of Consulting Psychology,* 1963, *27,* 324–330.

# Chapter 2

# The Psychological Value of Prepared Childbirth

THE BEGINNING OF A NEW LIFE always holds the potential to be an occasion of overwhelming joy. On learning of the pregnancy, parents may begin a series of preparations for the birth of the child. Parents may begin to plan for financial changes, prenatal care, and child care. The parents may also become anxious about what will happen when the time for the birth of the child arrives.

A variety of professionals, including physicians and psychologists, have argued that the preparation of the woman for childbirth represents an opportunity for the mother and a supportive partner, together with the appropriate health care team, to make the birth a pleasant physical and a positive psychological experience.

There has also been a resurgence of the layman's interest in preparation for childbirth. A visit to the local bookstore evidences the current popularity of Lamaze training, relaxation in childbirth, home births, birth without violence, and numerous other forms of parental preparation and involvement in the childbirth process. The research literature on the utility of prepared childbirth has grown greatly since the 1960s. Many published studies assess whether preparation for childbirth is beneficial and, if so, determine what the the benefits are.

The purpose of this chapter is to examine the currently available evidence on prepared childbirth. We will initially review the two most popular methods of preparation for childbirth. Then, we will turn our attention to the studies that have investigated the psychological utility of preparation for childbirth. In the third section of the chapter, we will evaluate the research methodologies used in these studies of childbirth preparation, suggest some ideas for future research, and offer a number of recommendations based on the current research evidence.

## LAMAZE AND DICK-READ: A BRIEF OVERVIEW

There are now available a host of different orientations and techniques to prepare parents for childbirth. For example, self-hypnosis (Kline & Guze, 1955), systematic desensitization (Kondas & Scetnicka, 1972) the psychoprophylactic method, and the Dick-Read method. The most popular methods are direct applications or derivatives of the systems developed by Lamaze and by Dick-Read. Since the research literature has focused on these two systems, we will briefly describe the main characteristics of each of the two approaches.

### The Dick-Read Method

Grantly Dick-Read, a British physician, developed his method (Dick-Read, 1953) of preparing women for childbirth based on the assumption that normal processes are ordinarily not painful, and birth should be no exception. Dick-Read reasoned that the severe pain reported by women during childbirth is a result of fear and apprehension, which are in turn derived from tradition. From Dick-Read's perspective, the attitudes and expectations communicated to women about childbirth, within the prevailing sociocultural climate, create a mental attitude that leads to tension and consequent inability to relax during childbirth. One need only recall the last time childbirth was portrayed in the media, with the woman writhing in pain and screaming, to understand what Dick-Read was suggesting. The fearful, tense woman, unable to relax, will experience a significantly greater amount of pain during childbirth. The basic assumption of Dick-Read's method is that if the pregnant woman can be taught to relax, and if her false notions about childbirth can be dispelled, then her experience in childbirth will be significantly less painful and significantly more pleasant.

The training of the gravid woman includes instruction in the female anatomy, the process of labor and delivery, and related areas of information relevant to childbirth. The instruction also includes exercises designed to improve general fitness for the birth process and instruction in breathing and relaxation exercises designed to be employed during labor to insure that the parturient will in fact remain relaxed. Dick-Read emphasized the desirability of minimal medical interference in the birth process. Hence, he viewed heavy sedation as generally undesirable.

### The Lamaze, or Psychoprophylactic, Method

This method for childbirth preparation was first developed by Russian physicians, was brought to France, and there was further developed by Ferdinand Lamaze. Although there is much similarity between the Lamaze method and the Dick-Read method, there are also some differences.

The psychoprophylactic method (which we will call PPM) is grounded theoretically in Pavlovian conditioning principles. The view is that pain in childbirth is exacerbated when the parturient interprets the bodily processes of labor as "pain" and reacts to these with moaning, groaning, and writhing. The PPM assumption is that before childbirth the woman can learn to substitute a different response to the contractions of labor; she can learn not to code the contractions as "pain" and, perhaps more important, she can learn to respond by engaging in behavior other than moaning and writhing.

The PPM classes are designed to provide information about the basic anatomy and processes of childbirth in order to correct erroneous ideas about labor and delivery. The classes also include exercises designed to improve general physical conditioning and breathing techniques designed to serve as positive alternative responses to the undesirable responses that most women would routinely give to the process of labor.

### Elements Common to Dick-Read and PPM

Although the methods are based on somewhat different perspectives, the Dick-Read and the PPM method of preparation for childbirth have much in common. In both there is the provision of information relevant to the childbirth process such as information about anatomy, contractions, and the stages of labor.

There is instruction in exercises that the pregnant woman can use to improve her general physical conditioning for labor and delivery. Both the PPM approach and the Dick-Read approach provide instruction in breathing techniques to be used during childbirth. Finally, both of these approaches assume and teach that the woman may be able to reduce pain by engaging in these activities. PPM instructors clearly and often tell their students that labor is a strenuous process and that some relief medication is quite acceptable. There may often be an implicit message, however, that less medication is better than more.

It is clear that the Dick-Read and PPM approaches share many elements. The two methods differ most in the theoretical conceptualization of the training programs but have a high degree of similarity in the actual methods used in preparing couples for childbirth. In the next section we will examine studies on these two major methods of preparing for childbirth to assess the effects of preparation for childbirth.

## THE EFFECTS OF PREPARATION FOR CHILDBIRTH

Although we recognize that any given PPM class or Dick-Read preparation will differ in specific emphases and in specific techniques taught, we feel that the commonalities are so great that we should examine these methods together. We will describe research studies that have investigated the effects of childbirth preparation on pain and discomfort, on the use of medication, on the duration of labor, and on the experience of positive emotional reactions to childbirth.

## Discomfort and Pain

Since the expected pain and discomfort of childbirth may be of utmost concern to the pregnant woman, research in this area may be most relevant both to the pregnant woman and to the professionals who will advise her about childbirth preparation.

Bergstrom-Walan (1963) obtained ratings by midwives who attended women in childbirth, along with ratings of anxiety in labor from the parturients themselves. Results indicated that the prepared mothers were rated less anxious both by the attending midwives and by themselves. Huttel, Mitchell, Fischer, and Meyer (1972) obtained ratings of the degree to which women complained and evidenced tension during labor and delivery. Women who had PPM preparation were rated as significantly less complaining and significantly less tense than women who did not have preparation for childbirth. Davenport-Slack and Boylan (1974) assessed body tenseness during delivery by analyzing ratings made by nurses who were unaware of whether or not the women had childbirth preparation. Nurses' rating of body tenseness was lower for women who had preparation than for those who did not. Fischer, Huttel, Mitchell, and Meyer (1972) obtained ratings of the degree to which the woman in labor was relaxed, showing self-control, and not screaming and tossing. Women who had PPM preparation were rated as significantly more relaxed and in control.

Tanzer (1968) and Tanzer and Block (1972) published a comparison of women who had PPM preparation for childbirth and a control group of women who did not. Women trained in PPM reported having significantly less pain during childbirth than did women in the control group. Bergstrom-Walan (1963) obtained ratings from the mothers themselves after parturition but before leaving the delivery room. The women were asked to rate, on a three-point scale, the amount of pain experienced. The women who had preparation reported experiencing significantly less pain than did women who had not wanted the preparation course or for whom the course was not available. Norr, Block, Charles, Meyering, and Meyers (1977) studied a sample of 249 women who were interviewed and who completed a questionnaire one to three days postpartum. PPM preparation was negatively correlated with reported pain in childbirth. Prepared women tended to report significantly less pain.

The results seem rather consistent. Women who have preparation for childbirth tend to report less pain and discomfort during childbirth, and they tend to be rated as less tense and anxious by attending medical personnel.

## Medication

One of the explicit goals of the Dick-Read approach is the reduction of medical "interference." Although PPM explicitly recognizes the possible need for medication during childbirth, the implicit norms of PPM groups may discourage the use of medication. Whether explicit or implicit, the norm of current methods of childbirth preparation is that where sedative or analgesic medication is concerned, less is better.

In 1953, Van Auken and Tomlinson reported a study in which they compared women who had attended Dick-Read classes with a group of women who had not. Although their description was somewhat incomplete by current standards, Van Auken and Tomlinson indicated that fewer women in the Dick-Read classes received general anesthesia during childbirth.

Davenport-Slack and Boylan (1974) reported a research project in which a group of women who chose PPM was compared with a group of women who chose not to participate in childbirth preparation classes. Significantly fewer of the trained women received general anesthesia.

Bergstrom-Walan (1963) conducted a study in which the reactions of four groups of women were examined: one group was asked to participate in a Dick-Read form of childbirth preparation and agreed; one group was asked but refused to participate in the childbirth preparation classes; one group volunteered for the preparation; and a fourth group did not have childbirth preparation classes available. Results indicated that there was not a difference in the amount of analgesic requested by the women. However, the results indicated that the women who had childbirth preparation received significantly less sedation than did women who did not have childbirth preparation.

Huttel and associates (1972) compared a group of women who had PPM preparation with a control group of randomly selected women who had not had preparation. The PPM group received significantly less medication during childbirth.

Fischer and associates (1972) compared a group of women who were persuaded to attend PPM classes with a group of women who did not attend PPM but who were cared for by the same staff during the same time period as the first group. A significantly greater percentage of the PPM group received no medication.

Three different groups of women were studied by Enkin, Smith, Dermer, and Emmett (1972). One group of women wanted PPM classes and attended them. A second group wanted PPM training but did not get it. A third group was comprised of women who did not ask for or attend PPM training, but these women were matched with those of other groups on age parity, and delivery date. The PPM group received significantly less analgesia.

A research project in which PPM training produced both less and more medication was reported by Scott and Rose (1976). These investigators compared a group of primiparas who had PPM preparation with a matched control group of women who were next to deliver at the same hospital, who were within five years of age of the first group, who had at least 37 weeks of gestation at parturition, and who had the same patient status (private or clinic patient) as the PPM women. Findings indicated that the PPM group had more women who received no medication at all during the first stage of labor, and significantly fewer women who received narcotics. On the other hand, women in the PPM group were more likely than women in the control group to receive a pudendal block for delivery.

Shapiro and Schmitt (1973) studied 200 primigravidas. One hundred had PPM preparation and the other 100 were a control group without preparation, who were consecutive admissions to the same hospital, and who had uncomplicated deliveries with vertex presentations. Results indicated that the PPM group was given smaller doses of narcotic medications per case. A greater percentage of women in the PPM group were given no narcotic medication at all, but the PPM women were more likely to receive pudendal anesthesia.

Laird and Hogan (1956) reported results similar to those described in the studies we have already reviewed. Women who had preparation for childbirth received less analgesia and a greater percentage of them received no medication at all during childbirth.

Up to this point we have reviewed studies that have shown that women prepared for childbirth tend to receive less medication. Not all of the available research has indicated such a difference.

Mandy, Mandy, Farkas, and Scher (1952) provided a somewhat incomplete description of the effects of preparing women for childbirth using the Dick-Read approach. The report was based on information provided to the authors by a colleague at London University. Mandy et al. indicated that there was no difference between prepared and unprepared women in the amount of analgesia received in childbirth.

In a study reported by Davis and Morrone (1962) primiparous women were interviewed prior to the twentieth week of pregnancy and asked whether they would like to participate in childbirth preparation. The description is deficient in the reporting of statistical summaries and tests, but the authors noted that there was no difference in the use of anesthesia for the two groups.

The two studies in which preparation for childbirth was found not to be related to a decreased use of anesthetics and/or analgesics are studies that lack extensive statistical descriptions and failed to report the appropriate statistical analyses. The other studies reviewed in this section indicated that childbirth preparation is related to the reduced use of medication in labor and delivery, especially to the reduced use of large amounts of medication.

It should be made clear that we are concluding only that childbirth preparation and the reduced utilization of certain medications during childbirth are related. We are not arguing that one causes the other. In a later section of this chapter we will discuss in more detail some of the possible variables that may be confounded with childbirth preparation in the current research. With specific reference to the use of medication in labor there is a variety of possible alternative explanations. Women prepared for childbirth may be less likely to request medication, physicians may be more likely to offer less medication to prepared women, or women who request childbirth preparation or who agree to participate in such programs may differ from women who do not. Regardless of the reason, however, women who are prepared for childbirth do have a lower probability of receiving general anesthetics or large amounts of analgesics during labor.

## Duration of Labor

Some studies have suggested that women who have preparation for childbirth may have shorter labors. Van Auken and Tomlinson (1953) reported that prepared women tended to have shorter labors than unprepared women. Bergstrom-Walan (1963), in a comparison of women prepared with the Dick-Read approach with groups of women who had not systematically prepared for childbirth, found that the prepared women had shorter labors. Shapiro and Schmitt (1973) found no difference between prepared and unprepared women in the duration of the second stage of labor; however, women who had PPM preparation had significantly shorter first stages of labor.

Several other studies, however, failed to find a relationship between preparation for childbirth and duration of labor. Mandy et al. (1952) reported that duration of labor for women trained for childbirth was not different from that of untrained women. Davis and Morrone (1962), although they did not report their statistics in detail, indicated that there was no relationship between labor duration and preparation for childbirth in the sample they studied. Davenport-Slack and Boylan (1974) also reported similar results.

Zax, Sameroff, and Farnum (1975) compared women who had PPM training with women who had not had PPM training. They reported that duration of labor was not reliably related to preparation for childbirth. Scott and Rose (1976) reported similar results when they compared two groups of primiparas, only one of which had PPM preparation.

Huttel et al. (1972) and Fischer et al. (1972) both reported a trend suggesting that PPM preparation is related to shorter duration of labor, but in both studies the observed differences favoring PPM were not statistically reliable.

The available data, then, seem to suggest that if preparation for childbirth affects duration of labor at all, it may shorten labor. However, the major portion of the available research evidence suggests that preparation for childbirth will not be related to labor duration at all.

Perhaps of all the factors reviewed, duration of labor may be the most difficult to measure reliably. Since most women are usually not under the direct observation of medical personnel when labor begins, it may be difficult to establish exactly the time at which labor started. Furthermore, it is possible that preparation for childbirth may lead the parturient to feel more confident in her ability to deal with contractions, and she may be somewhat slower in contacting her physician or in going to the hospital. One conclusion is clear from the available data. There is no indication that preparation increases the duration of labor. The most frequent finding is that duration of labor has no relationship to childbirth preparation; if there is a relationship, it will be a tendency for labor to be somewhat shorter with preparation.

## Positive Emotions

The literature on natural childbirth and prepared childbirth often refers to childbirth as a highly positive emotional experience, an experience that is intensely meaningful to women giving birth. We will now examine the handful of studies that have attempted to evaluate the relationship between preparation and the experience of positive emotional reactions during childbirth.

Tanzer (1968) and Tanzer and Block (1972) noted that women with PPM preparation reported having more positive emotions during parturition than did a comparison group of women. Enkin et al. (1972) asked women to respond to a questionnaire four to six months postpartum. This study included a control group of women who wanted childbirth preparation classes but did not receive them. Results indicated that women who had PPM preparation for childbirth had significantly more positive recollections about labor, delivery, and the overall childbirth experience. Norr et al. (1977) found that participation in PPM training was significantly correlated with reported enjoyment of the childbirth experience. Women who had PPM preparation spontaneously mentioned feelings of joy during childbirth and gave more positive ratings of the experience. Doering and Entwisle (1975) contacted women postpartum and interviewed participants in their homes. Women who had prepared for childbirth were contacted and a comparison group of untrained women was obtained through referrals from the other participants. Prepared women tended to report being significantly more aware during childbirth and they tended to evidence a significantly more positive attitude toward the childbirth experience.

The conclusion suggested by the studies available is that preparation is significantly related to more positive recollections about the childbirth experience. Again we are faced with a problem that we will discuss in more detail later: what causes the relationship between preparation and a positive experience in childbirth? The available studies suggest the relationship is there, but the data have some deficiencies that make causal inferences very tenuous. Before turning to an evaluation of the research studies we have reviewed, let us briefly summarize what the main findings seem to be.

## Summary of Findings

The pain, discomfort, and tension experienced by women in childbirth tend to be less intense for women who have had preparation. Most of the studies relied on recollections about the birth experience, but the studies that included ratings by other persons reported results congruent with the self-report studies.

Although not all studies reviewed obtained significant results, the available evidence seems to suggest that women who attend prepared childbirth programs are less likely to receive general anesthesia, tend to receive smaller doses of analgesic, and are more likely to receive no medication. Some recent studies have indicated that prepared women may be more likely to receive pudendal anesthesia.

Findings regarding the duration of labor suggest that childbirth preparation and duration of labor tend to be unrelated. In the few studies in which a relationship was reported, prepared women tended to have shorter labors.

Finally, although few studies have examined the positive reactions experienced by women in childbirth, the available findings suggest that women who have training are more likely to describe the birth experience more positively and recall it more favorably than are untrained women.

# AN EVALUATION AND DIRECTIONS FOR FUTURE RESEARCH

Perhaps the most important methodological issue in the series of studies examined here is the use of appropriate control groups of women who have not had preparation for childbirth. The ideal method of placing subjects in different conditions is the random assignment of participants to various conditions. The study by Huttel et al. (1972) is the only one that described its method of subject assignment as random. Any researcher who has attempted to conduct research in a clinical setting knows the practical restrictions that research in such a setting entails. Random assignment is often impossible because of institutional constraints, and random assignment of participants to a control group often raises serious ethical implications. Although it is understandable that research on prepared childbirth has not included random assignment of subjects on a wide scale, this failure must still temper the degree to which we can unambiguously evaluate the contributions of prepared childbirth.

Although the ideal of random assignment of subjects to groups has not been met, almost all studies reviewed, especially the more recent ones, included a comparison group. The typical comparison group has been an untrained group. There are many possible differences, however, between women who participate in childbirth preparation and those who do not in terms of religious preference, educational level, and occupation, for example (Leonard, 1973; Ostrum, 1972). If the women differ on such dimensions, findings with respect to pain and medication may result from those variables and not specifically the preparation or lack of it. One variable that is necessary to rule out as a possible causal factor is the desire to participate in childbirth preparation. At least three studies have included comparison groups designed to control for the desire to participate (Bergstrom-Walan, 1963; Enkin et al., 1972; Huttel et al., 1972). Other studies have included matched controls: the women prepared for childbirth were matched on certain variables with a comparison group of unprepared women (Scott & Rose, 1976; Shapiro & Schmitt, 1973). Still other research reports have relied on a comparison group of unprepared women neither randomly assigned nor systematically matched on a variety of dimensions with a prepared group (Davenport-Slack & Boylan, 1974; Davis & Morrone, 1962; Fischer et al., 1972; Laird & Hogan, 1956; Mandy et al., 1952; Tanzer, 1968; Zax et al., 1975). Finally, at least two studies were correlational studies (Doering & Entwisle, 1975; Norr et al., 1977).

A number of possible confounding variables should increase our caution in attributing the cause of the summarized findings to preparation for childbirth. We are not suggesting that differences we have concluded to exist between prepared and unprepared groups do not exist. The issue is whether we can confidently attribute such differences to the preparation. Our causal inferences should be tempered by the following potential confounding variables: the presence of the husband or another coach during labor, the expectation that childbirth preparation will help the woman deal positively with the stress of childbirth, the attitudes and expectations of medical personnel regarding the labor of women who have prepared for childbirth, the possibility that women who accept or choose to attend childbirth preparation programs may differ in many ways from those who do not, and the provision of accurate information about what will happen during labor and delivery. The currently available studies do not permit us to rule out some of these confounding variables as possible causal agents that produce the differences in labor experience between parturients who have had and those who have not had childbirth training.

However, on the positive side, at least two factors favor preparation as a possible cause. First, the three studies that included strong controls for some of these potential confounds (Bergstrom-Walan, 1963; Enkin et al., 1972; Huttel et al., 1972) reported reliable positive effects for childbirth preparation. Bergstrom-Walan (1963) found that trained women experienced less pain and discomfort and received less sedation than did untrained women. Enkin et al. (1972) reported that trained women received less medication and recalled the birth experience in more positive terms. Huttel et al. (1972) reported that women with PPM preparation had lower ratings of tension and discomfort during labor and received less medication than women without PPM preparation. Second, the comparison groups used in other studies have included varying degrees of experimental control, and those studies also have suggested positive effects for childbirth preparation.

Our conclusion regarding the research methodologies employed in studies of childbirth preparation is that it is not possible to say unambiguously that childbirth preparation produced the observed differences. But, the studies in which alternative explanations were minimized still showed favorable effects of prepared childbirth. Hence, while maintaining a certain healthy skepticism about the specific causal factors, we suggest that in spite of the limitations of available research, preparation for childbirth does appear to have positive effects.

Programs preparing couples for childbirth involve a number of specific components including breathing techniques, physical exercises, group discussions, information about delivery, and the involvement of supportive persons. Current research does not allow us to evaluate the relative importance of each of these specific factors in producing the differences between those women who prepare for childbirth and those who do not. An important task for further research in this area would seem to be the examination of the relative contribution of each of the various components of the PPM program: comparisons of a program that included information on the processes of labor and delivery, for example, with a program that did not. Such investigation would enhance the potential effectiveness of childbirth preparation programs by identifying the important components of training.

Future research could also profitably examine individual differences in both husband and wife that may improve the benefits from preparation. Individual differences in such areas as state and trait anxiety (Spielberger, 1971; Zax et al., 1975) and related measures may be useful avenues for investigation. Understanding of such relationships might allow prediction of women who may need more medication, providing more accurate identification of the woman who may require more support and assistance during labor and delivery.

## SOME RECOMMENDATIONS

Unless further research in the area clearly indicates that a particular element of childbirth preparation programs is not essential, we would like to recommend the following procedures.

## Information

The pregnant woman and her partner should be offered specific, clear, and unambiguous information about the anatomy, mechanisms, signs, and course of labor and childbirth. We use the word "offered" because some women may choose not to learn about parturition, and it may be best not to force information on them. Information should be available in written form both from the consulting physician or other health professional and from childbirth preparation classes. Information in written form is easy to locate: pamphlets may be available gratis from a variety of sources and there are many books currently available that provide excellent information, among them *Our Bodies, Ourselves* (Boston Women's Health Book Collective, 1976) and *Pregnancy, Birth, and the Newborn Baby* (Boston Children's Medical Center, 1972).

The attending physician should be available for questions from the patient, should encourage questions, and should answer them clearly and truthfully. Again, the patient should determine how much information is transmitted. The physician should be alert to the patient's needs, providing the level of information that she requests. Although perhaps more important for primigravidas, a brief description of the particular procedures to be used in labor and delivery should be included. Any peculiarities of delivery rooms and labor areas should be dealt with long before labor begins. The physician and patient should also make explicit their expectations about procedures during labor and delivery, and we think the physician should be open to requests from patients regarding such areas as medication and presence of the husband.

Well-staffed programs in childbirth preparation can be a highly beneficial resource for the pregnant woman and her partner. The semi-structured format used by some Lamaze programs, for example, provides a systematic presentation of information about childbirth in a group atmosphere in which mutual support can occur and in which individual requests for information can be accommodated.

## Involvement of the Husband

Several years ago, one of our colleagues told his wife's obstetrician that he would like to be with his wife in the labor and delivery areas of the hospital at the birth of their first child. As our colleague related the incident, the physician hesitated a bit before answering and then indicated that he could not allow our colleague to be present since husbands who are present at their wives' delivery run a very high risk of subsequently developing erectile dysfunction. Whether or not the physician's response was flippant, he remained opposed to the husband's being with his wife during childbirth.

Not all objections are facetious. Some physicians may be concerned about increased problems in maintaining a sterile environment, others may be wary of the husband's presence in case complications should develop, and others may simply find the husband's presence inconvenient. In spite of the objections raised we feel that medical personnel should not only permit attendance of, but also provide support for, the husband who wishes to participate in the childbirth process with his wife. (Although we use the word "husband," we are not suggesting that in order for a woman's partner to be helpful he must be legally married to the parturient.)

The presence of a supporting and helpful partner may prove beneficial to the woman giving birth. Tanzer (1968) and Tanzer and Block (1972) reported that all women who had joyful and rapturous childbirth experiences had their husbands present. Since he is not directly experiencing the physical stress of labor, the husband may be able to provide accurate feedback about contractions and labor duration. He is also able to provide comfort and support for his wife throughout the childbirth experience.

The presence of the husband during childbirth may be a beneficial experience for him, too. We are unaware of any research data that suggest that the husband's presence is psychologically damaging for him. On the other hand, some data suggest that husbands who are present during labor and delivery may have a more positive reaction to the birth than husbands who are not present (Cronenwett & Newmark, 1974; Henneborn & Cogan, 1975). However, just as with PPM training for the woman alone, forcing the father into PPM labor room or delivery room participation is unwise.

Our feeling is that the health care specialist should actively support the couple who want the husband to participate in the process of welcoming a new person to our midst.

## Breathing and Relaxation Techniques

As we have previously indicated, the current data do not permit an unambiguous inference of the specific elements responsible for the more positive birth experience that prepared women have. However, we think that the breathing and relaxation techniques are useful in labor and delivery. Even if the effect of these measures may be largely placebo (i.e. nonspecific), they still seem to serve a useful function to the woman in labor. Participation in a childbirth preparation program that teaches techniques to be used during parturition is a useful endeavor for the pregnant woman and her partner.

## Support from Health Care Professionals

Our final recommendation is that attending physicians, nurses, midwives, and other persons be supportive of the woman during labor. This recommendation is superfluous in most instances since professionals generally are supportive in their interactions with patients. We are suggesting that individuals involved in assisting women during pregnancy and childbirth be open to the interest that many women have in taking an active part in giving birth. The woman and her husband should be encouraged in their efforts at preparation, and the woman should be supported in her efforts to implement her learning during the childbirth process.

In their zeal to be advocates of childbirth preparation many individuals may exaggerate the benefits, thus leading some health professionals to become hesitant about believing any claims for such training. Our personal experiences with childbirth preparation have been positive, and we think the available evidence also supports the utility of childbirth preparation. It is not a panacea; peak experiences during childbirth may very well not be the rule; and all of the claims made for childbirth preparation are not necessarily correct. But childbirth preparation may lead to less tension and pain, to less medication during labor and delivery, and to a more positive emotional response to the experience of birth. It is possible that other benefits may accrue to infants born to prepared mothers. Improved Apgar scores may be associated with decreased analgesia, anesthetics, and sedative medication. In addition, immediate post partum maternal infant bonding described in chapter 7 may also be facilitated in the alert, functional mother who has successfully utilized PPM technique with less medication. There is increasing evidence that important mother child interaction occurs during the first hours or even minutes of the infant's life. Desirable adaptive bonding early after birth may be facilitated by preparation for childbirth. Attending medical personnel should be open to prepared childbirth programs which provide greater involvement of the parents in the arrival of their child.

## REFERENCES


BEAN, C. A. *Methods of childbirth*. New York: Doubleday, 1972.

BERGSTROM-WALAN, M. Efficacy of education for childbirth. *Journal of Psychosomatic Research*, 1963, *7*, 131-146.

BLANFIELD, A. Conflicts created by childbirth methodologies. In N. Morris (ed.), *Psychosomatic medicine in obstetrics and gynecology*. Basel: S. Karger, 1972.

Boston Children's Medical Center. *Pregnancy, birth, and the newborn baby*. New York: Delacorte, 1972.

Boston Women's Health Book Collective. *Our bodies, ourselves* (2d ed.). New York: Simon & Schuster, 1976.

BULMAN, N. W. The psychological aspect of obstetrics. *Nursing Times*, 1937, *32*, 1044-1047.

BUXTON, C. L. *A study of psychophysical methods for relief of childbirth pain*. Philadelphia: Saunders, 1962.

CASTALLO, M. A. Preparing parents for parenthood. *Journal of the American Medical Association*, 1958, *166*, 1970-1973.

CHABON, I. *Awake and aware*. New York: Delacorte, 1966.

CHERTOK, L. Psychosomatic methods of preparation for childbirth. *American Journal of Obstetrics and Gynecology*, 1967, *98*, 698-703.

——. *Motherhood and personality: psychosomatic aspects of childbirth*. Philadelphia: Lippincott, 1969.

COGAN, R. Use of relaxation and breathing after labor contractions begin. *Birth and the Family Journal,* 1974, *1,* 16–18.

CRONENWETT, L. R., and NEWMARK, L. C. Fathers' responses to childbirth. *Nursing Research,* 1974, *23,* 210–217.

DAVENPORT-SLACK, B., and BOYLAN, C. H. Psychological correlates of childbirth pain. *Psychosomatic Medicine,* 1974, *36,* 215–223.

DAVIS, C. D., and MORRONE, F. A. An objective evaluation of a prepared childbirth program. *American Journal of Obstetrics and Gynecology,* 1962, *84,* 1196–1206.

DICK-READ, G. *Childbirth without fear.* New York: Harper, 1953.

DOERING, S. G. & ENTWISLE, D. R. Preparation during pregnancy and ability to cope with labor and delivery. *American Journal of Orthopsychiatry,* 1975, *45,* 825–837.

ENKIN, M. W., SMITH, S. L., DERMER, S. W., and EMMETT, J. O. An adequately controlled study of the effectiveness of PPM training. In N. Morris (ed.), *Psychosomatic medicine in obstetrics and gynecology.* Basel: S. Karger, 1972.

ESTY, G. P. Natural childbirth: a word from a mother. *American Journal of Nursing,* 1969, *69,* 1453–1454.

EWY, D., and EWY, R. *Preparation for childbirth: a Lamaze guide.* Boulder: Pruett, 1970.

FISCHER, W. M., HUTTEL, F. A., MITCHELL, I., and MEYER, A. E. The efficacy of the psychoprophylactic method of prepared childbirth. In N. Morris (ed.), *Psychosomatic Medicine in Obstetrics and Gynecology.* Basel: S. Karger, 1972.

FREEDMAN, L. Z., REDLICH, F. C., ERON, L. D., and JACKSON, E. B. Training for childbirth: remembrance of labor. *Psychosomatic Medicine,* 1952, *14* 439–452.

HENNEBORN, W. J., and COGAN, R. The effect of husband participation on reported pain and probability of medication during labor and birth. *Journal of Psychosomatic Research,* 1975, *19,* 215–222.

HOTT, J. R. An investigation of the relationship between psychoprophylaxis in childbirth and changes in self-concept of the participant husband and his concept of his wife. *Dissertations Abstracts International,* 1972, *33*(1-B), 296–297.

HUTTEL, F. A., MITCHELL, I., FISCHER, W. M., and MEYER, A. E. A quantitative evaluation of psychoprophylaxis in childbirth. *Journal of Psychosomatic Research,* 1972, *16,* 81–92.

KLINE, M. V., and GUZE, H. Self-hypnosis in childbirth. *International Journal of Clinical and Experimental Hypnosis,* 1955, *3,* 142–147.

KLUSMAN, L. E. Reduction of pain in childbirth by the alleviation of anxiety during pregnancy. *Journal of Consulting and Clinical Psychology,* 1975, *43,* 162–165.

KONDAS, O., and SCETNICKA, B. Systematic desensitization as a method of preparation for childbirth. *Journal of Behavior Therapy and Experimental Psychiatry,* 1972, *3,* 51–54.

LAIRD, M. D., and HOGAN, M. An elective program of preparation for childbirth at the Sloan Hospital for Women. *American Journal of Obstetrics and Gynecology,* 1956, *72,* 641–647.

LEONARD, R. F. Evaluation of selection tendencies of patients preferring prepaid childbirth. *Obstetrics and Gynecology,* 1973, *42,* 371–377.

MANDY, A. J., MANDY, T. E., FARKAS, R., and SCHER, E. Is natural childbirth natural? *Psychosomatic Medicine,* 1952, *14,* 431–438.

MCCALL, J. O. The Lamaze lament. *Transactions of the Pacific Coast Obstetrical and Gynecological Society,* 1975, *42,* 127–132.

MCNEIL, A. T. The Soviet or psychoprophylactic method of painless childbirth. *Cerebral Palsy Bulletin,* 1961, *3,* 159–166.

MILLER, J. S. Childbirth: progress in dignity. *Journal of Humanistic Psychology,* 1971, *1,* 85–92.

NETTELBLADT, P., FAGERSTRÖM, C. F., and UDDENBERG, N. The significance of reported childbirth pain. *Journal of Psychosomatic Research,* 1976, *20,* 215–222.

NORR, K. L., BLOCK, C. R., CHARLES, A., MEYERING, S., and MEYERS, E. Explaining pain and enjoyment in childbirth. *Journal of Health and Social Behavior,* 1977, *18,* 260–275.

OSTRUM, A. E. Psychological factors influencing women's choice of childbirth procedure. *Dissertation Abstracts International,* 1972, *33*(5-B), 2353.

ROSENGREN, W. R. Some social psychological aspects of delivery room difficulties. *Journal of Nervous and Mental Disease,* 1961, *132,* 515–521.

SCOTT, J. R., and ROSE, N. B. Effect of psychoprophylaxis on labor and delivery in primiparas. *New England Journal of Medicine,* 1976, *294,* 1205–1207.

SHAPIRO, H. I., and SCHMITT, L. G. Evaluation of the psychoprophylactic method of childbirth in the primigravida. *Connecticut Medicine,* 1973, *37,* 341–343.

SPIELBERGER, C. D. (Ed.) *Anxiety: Current trends in theory and research.* New York: Academic Press, 1971.

SWARTZ, R. A father's view. *Children Today,* 1977, *6,* 14–17.

TANZER, D. Natural childbirth: pain or peak experience? *Psychology Today,* 1968, *2*(5), 17–21.

TANZER, D., and BLOCK, J. L. *Why natural childbirth.* New York: Doubleday, 1972.

THOMPSON, L. J. Attitudes of primiparae as observed in a prenatal clinic. *Mental Hygiene,* 1942, *26,* 243–256.

THOMS, H., and KARLOVSKY, E. D. Two thousand deliveries under a training for childbirth program: a statistical survey and commentary. *American Journal of Obstetrics and Gynecology,* 1954, *68,* 279–284.

ULIN, P. R. Changing techniques in psychoprophylactic preparation for childbirth. *American Journal of Nursing,* 1968, *68,* 2586–2591.

VAN AUKEN, W. B., and TOMLINSON, D. R. An appraisal of patient training for childbirth. *American Journal of Obstetrics and Gynecology,* 1953, *66,* 100–105.

WINDWER, C. Relationship among prospective parents' locus of control, social desirability, and choice of psychoprophylaxis. *Nursing Research,* 1977, *26,* 96–99.

YAHIA, C., and ULIN, P. R. Preliminary experience with a psychophysical program of preparation for childbirth. *American Journal of Obstetrics and Gynecology,* 1965, *93,* 942–949.

ZAX, M., SAMEROFF, A. J., and FARNUM, J. E. Childbirth education, maternal attitudes, and delivery. *American Journal of Obstetrics and Gynecology,* 1975, *123,* 185–190.

ZUCKERMAN, M., NURNBERGER, J. I., GARDINER, S. H., VANDIVEER, J. M., BARRETT, B. H., and DEN BREEIJEN, A. Psychological correlates of somatic complaints in pregnancy and difficulty in childbirth. *Journal of Consulting Psychology,* 1963, *27,* 324–330.

# Chapter 3

# Psychological Responses to Terminated Pregnancy

ABORTION IS AN ISSUE that is highly charged emotionally and has only within the last two decades become the focus of scientific investigation in the United States. Prior to the liberalization of the Colorado state law regarding abortion in 1967, few publications in the United States dealt with the issue of a woman's emotional reaction to abortion. Those publications that dealt with reactions to abortion were typically opinions, and very little clinical or experimental data were reported. Following the liberalization of the Colorado law, the issue of abortion became more public, and several investigators in the United States began to look at a woman's psychological reaction to abortion. This chapter will examine women's reactions to abortion.

First, however, the terminology needs to be clarified. This chapter will focus on several types of abortion: spontaneous abortions, habitual abortions, medically necessitated abortions, and therapeutic abortions. The *spontaneous abortion, or miscarriage,* is the spontaneous loss of the fetus during the first trimester. This type of abortion is accidentally caused, is non-recurrent, and is usually of unknown etiology. Both maternal factors (pathological anatomy and physiology of the reproductive tract) and embryonic factors, (most commonly chromosomal abnormalities) are cited as likely causes. The *habitual aborter,* on the other hand, is a woman who is successively unsuccessful in her gestational experience and is defined in the literature as a woman who has had three consecutive spontaneous abortions. There are several types of abortion that are induced by physicians. The first that will be described in this chapter is the *medically necessitated abortion.* The majority of studies describing a woman's reactions to a medically necessitated abortion include abortions performed because of the high risk of the physical health of the mother, as well as abortions performed because the mother, and therefore the fetus, have been exposed to a disease such as rubella, which is likely to cause significant malformations or deformaties in the fetus. A medically necessitated abortion would also include those abortions that are determined to be medically necessary because of genetic factors. The health of the mother is not an issue in these abortions; rather, it is the probable health of the fetus. Amniocentesis (needed aspiration of a small amount of amniotic fluid) is often used to determine whether or not the child has been affected by the genetically transmitted disease; however, in some cases, the disease cannot be diagnosed via amniocentesis. Since the sex of the child can be determined by amniocentesis and since some genetic diseases are sex-linked, in some cases abortions are performed because of genetic reasons when the probability of the disease's being transmitted, because of the sex of the child, is high. Finally, *therapeutic abortions* are those abortions performed because of potential detriment to the mental health of the mother. It must be made clear that following the liberalization of the 1967 Colorado state law, abortions became more available to less seriously psychiatrically disturbed women in several states, Colorado and New York being two. Thus, until the Supreme Court decision of 1973, which determined that abortion in the first trimester is the decision of the woman, all women obtaining abortions had to do so because of the stated possibility of risk to their emotional and psychological health. Until 1967 a woman had to pass extremely stringent criteria in order to obtain a "therapeutic abortion." However, with the liberalization in attitudes toward abortion, the criteria became less and less stringent so that in 1971, 1972, and 1973, the majority of women who were allowed to obtain therapeutic abortions would probably have been denied these abortions in earlier years. Thus, the section on therapeutic abortions includes a very heterogeneous group of women. There is no way, however, to sort out those women who have serious psychological disturbances from those whose disturbances relate specifically to an unwanted pregnancy. For this reason all the studies between 1967 and the 1973 Supreme Court decision have been grouped under the term "therapeutic abortions." Following the Supreme Court decision, women were allowed to obtain elective abortions; that is, any woman requesting an abortion in the first trimester was able to obtain one. The reaction of women to elective abortions will not be covered in this chapter. Reviews of elective abortions are available elsewhere (e.g., Calhoun, Selby, & King, 1976).

## SPONTANEOUS ABORTION

The literature regarding psychological sequelae to spontaneous abortion is sparse and many studies do not distinguish spontaneous from habitual aborters. A few studies have addressed these issues.

Simon, Rothman, Goff, and Senturia (1969) compared 32 spontaneous aborters to 46 women obtaining therapeutic abortions. In this study therapeutic abortions included abortions obtained for a variety of indications: medical illness, psychiatric illness, and possible fetal damage. Each woman was interviewed by one of the authors in a semistructured interview and completed a special questionnaire, the Minnesota Multiphasic Personality Inventory (MMPI) and the Loevinger Family Problems Scale. This was a retrospective study and information obtained from hospital records was also used. The women who had spontaneous abortions were found to be more likely to be depressed at the time of the abortion (13 of 32) and depression was found more frequently in those women whose pregnancies were planned than in those with unplanned pregnancies. Guilt was relatively infrequent (22%) in spontaneous aborters as opposed to therapeutic aborters (35%) and appeared to be correlated with the presence of psychiatric illness in women in both groups.

Differences between MMPI scores of spontaneous and therapeutic aborters were noted, as well as differences from a normative group. Both the therapeutic aborters and the spontaneous aborters had higher scores on the Pd Scale (psychopathic deviate) and lower scores on the M-F Scale (masculinity-feminity) than did the normative group. The normative group scores were obtained by Hathaway and Briggs (1957) from a large normal population of women. Although the scores of both groups differed significantly from the norm group in the direction of psychopathology, only 2 women in the spontaneous abortion group and 17 in the therapeutic abortion group had scores in the deviant range. The elevated scores on the Pd Scale would suggest the possibility of greater unconventionality and more rebelliousness, and the lower scores on the M-F Scale suggest that both groups endorse items that are exaggerations of traditional beliefs about femininity.

The typical immediate reaction evidenced by the spondaneous abortion group was transient grief. Those women who also evidenced guilt and depression postabortion were more likely to experience psychiatric difficulties later. At the time of the interview 62.5% of the spontaneous abortion group had a diagnosable psychiatric disorder as opposed to 70% of the therapeutic abortion group. By itself the difference in frequency is misleading, however, since the authors reported that psychiatric disorders were much more severe in the therapeutic abortion group (there were no psychoses in the spontaneous abortion group). Additionally, the authors viewed the psychiatric problems of the therapeutic abortion group as part of a chronic pattern, whereas difficulties in the spontaneous abortion group seemed more clearly related to the abortion.

Depressed feelings or feelings of disappointment following a spontaneous abortion have been frequently noted (Freundt, 1964; Malmquist, Kaij, & Nilsson, 1969; Simon et al., 1969). Corney and Horton (1974) presented a clinical description of one woman suffering from pathological grief following a spontaneous abortion. They contrasted grief, a state of emotional suffering caused by the loss of a loved person through death, with pathological grief, an inability to mourn the deceased person appropriately, which leads to chronic preoccupation and sadness. The description of the case is interesting and serves to illustrate several factors that may increase the likelihood of a pathological grief reaction following a spontaneous abortion. Factors such as an unplanned pregnancy, a pregnancy about which the woman is ambivalent, or a pregnancy in which the father is emotionally uninvolved or rejecting may predispose a woman to a pathological grief reaction. The unexpected loss of the pregnancy, especially in an atmosphere not conducive to expressions of grief and sadness (such as a hospital ward), may precipitate difficulties specifically by hindering the mourning of the loss at the appropriate time. This inability to mourn then results in chronic sadness and/or depression. Corney and Horton hypothesized that the women in the Simon, et al. (1969) study who continued to be depressed for a year or more might be having a distorted or prolonged grief reaction.

Malmquist, Kaij, and Nilsson (1969) compared 84 women who had had one or more spontaneous abortions prior to pregnancy with 84 women having no such difficulties. The two groups were matched in age, parity, marital status, socioeconomic status, and length of marriage. The results of questionnaires showed that the spontaneous aborters had more bleeding two months postpartum, more genital pain early postpartum, and more babies with problems. From a psychiatric point of view the spontaneous abortion group was more heterogeneous as these women reported either no symptoms or many symptoms (more than nine). Only two psychiatric symptoms discriminated the two groups. The spontaneous aborters reported more unsteadiness, or vertigo, and more depression. Additionally, more women who had had spontaneous abortions had symptoms during the year prior to pregnancy. The finding concerning depression in the year prior to pregnancy perhaps reflected the grief reaction of these women to a spontaneous abortion preceding the pregnancy. Whether the reported symptoms were part of an immediate grief reaction or part of a more chronic depression, these results confirmed the findings of Simon et al. (1969). These authors noted a high frequency of both immediate grief reactions and chronic depression in women following a spontaneous abortion.

In summary, the literature regarding spontaneous abortions seems to suggest the possibility of a short-term grief reaction to the loss of the child, as well as a more prolonged depressive state in the months following the spontaneous abortion. The extent to which these reactions are part of a pathological grief reaction to the loss of the fetus or a more personal loss of self-esteem and self-worth caused by failure to have carried the pregnancy to term remains a question.

## HABITUAL ABORTION

The habitual aborter is defined as a woman who has had three or more successive spontaneous abortions. Many different regimens—hormones, vitamins, surgery, bed rest, and sexual abstinence—have been used successfully with habitual aborters; however, none is effective consistently. Javert (1954), in utilizing a treatment program of vitamins, employed psychotherapy as an adjunct and became increasingly impressed with the apparent emotional factors involved with habitual aborters. He formulated a stress-related mechanism to explain the onset of premature labor. Earlier, Squire and Dunbar (1946) had regarded the abortion habit as similar to accident-proneness and argued that psychotherapy might break the habit.

Mann (1959) developed a clinic for habitual aborters in order to evaluate these women psychiatrically. Only women who had experienced three consecutive spontaneous abortions and who had no apparent physical causes for the spontaneous abortions were seen. Each woman was interviewed preconceptionally with her husband and the psychiatric orientation of the program was explained. An average of three to four interviews over a period of two months occurred before the woman became pregnant. According to Mann the typical reaction to pregnancy was anxiety and increased dependency, and each woman continued to be seen and given reassurance and support about her pregnancy. Once quickening occurred women talked more about the unborn child during the interview.

In analyzing these interviews, Mann described the habitual aborter as a very dependent personality who is overinvolved with her own mother and unable to relate adequately to her husband. In his view each pregnancy is an attempt by the women to progress to a more independent and mature life. However, as her anxiety increases, the woman regresses, and she aborts. Spontaneous abortion allows her to retreat from maturity. In his view supportive psychotherapy that allows a term birth can be a very growth producing experience for these women.

Published reports of the first 16 months of Mann's study included 65 habitual aborters who were seen, psychiatrically evaluated, and followed. A total of 24 patients either had carried to term or had aborted, 18 were in various stages of pregnancy, and 23 were still in the preconception phase. The 24 patients had had a total of 90 previous pregnancies, 84 of which had ended in miscarriage. Thus, 93.3% of their pregnancies had ended in spontaneous abortion before treatment. During treatment 20 delivered normal living infants; 4 spontaneously aborted (16.6%).

Grimm (1962) reported on the psychological test results of several women who participated in the Cornell project on habitual aborters (Mann, 1959). An experimental group of 61 habitual aborters and a comparison group of 35 women who had no history of spontaneous abortion were subjects in part one of the study. Of the comparison group 17 were "normal" pregnant women who were tested before the fourth month of pregnancy; 18 were nonpregnant women referred for a gynecological difficulty of possible psychosomatic origin. The women in the habitual abortion group were not pregnant but were planning to become pregnant. There were no significant differences in age at marriage, education level, IQ, race, religion, or socioeconomic factors between the habitual aborters and the comparison group; however, the habitual aborter was an average of four years older.

The women in both groups were all given a Wechsler-Bellevue Intelligence Scale, a Rorschach, and the Thematic Apperception Test (TAT). The abortion-prone women performed more poorly on the picture arrangement subtest of the Wechsler-Bellevue. The function theorized to underlie this subtest is the ability to size up a social situation utilizing visual cues and to plan and anticipate correctly. Other differences were noted on the Rorschach protocols. The abortion-prone women gave a far greater number of color-form than of form-color responses and a larger number of popular responses. Grimm theorized that the first difference suggested a lack of control of emotions and a tendency to act out conflicts, whereas the second suggested excessive social adaptability and conformity. The content of the percepts on the Rorschach was evaluated and aborters were found to have significantly more responses indicating indirect hostility and tension concerning its expression. (A response suggesting indirect hostility would be a percept in which an underlying concern with aggression or destruction is reflected; e.g, weapons, claws, or explosions.) On the TAT the frequency of each type of theme—hostility, helping, or guilt—was scored for each card and summed across all cards. The aborters were found to have a significantly higher frequency of helping and guilt themes; there were no differences with regard to aggression. These scores suggest that habitual aborters have stronger feelings of dependency and greater proneness to guilt feelings. A total of 10 test indicators across all tests were found to discriminate between the two groups.

Grimm (1962) characterized the women in the habitual abortion group as dependent and overly compliant women who cannot openly express anger and/or frustration in stressful or demanding situations for fear of rejection and guilt. Instead, they remain compliant and tension increases in these emotionally reactive women until they have a psychosomatic reaction (abortion) that relieves the tension. This formulation is similar to those expressed by Mann (1959) and by Weil and Tupper (1960).

Thirty-two of the 61 aborters described in part one of the Grimm (1962) study were followed after becoming pregnant and were retested after the thirty-fifth week of pregnancy. The thirty-fifth week was chosen because the fetus was viable and the patient was considered to have lost the original symptom of abortion-proneness. Twenty-two women successfully carried to term and five aborted. Thus, for this group of 27 women psychotherapy appeared to be a very efficacious procedure. For the 22 success cases

(81%), test results from the readministration of Rorschach, TAT, and Wechsler-Bellevue were compared to the results from the original testing of each woman. Grimm noted a total of seven test indicators that changed significantly from one administration to the next. Four of these seven had been found to discriminate between the aborters and the controls in part one of the study, and all changes were in the direction of the control group (regression to the mean?). Following therapy and success in carrying the fetus to 35 weeks the test results suggested change in the direction of greater emotional control, less buildup of tension in relationship to feelings of hostility, and less guilt. Three additional changes were noted by Grimm: the women gave fewer responses, showed less bodily preoccupation, and had more neutral content in their responses.

Grimm did not argue that these psychological variables are the cause of habitual abortion; rather, she viewed these results as suggesting a certain constellation of personality characteristics that typifies the majority of women prone to habitual abortion.

Tupper, Moya, Stewart, Weil, and Gray (1957) did a descriptive study of 100 women they classified as habitual aborters; however, they did not separate habitual from spontaneous aborters. The 100 patients were given clinical interviews and a questionnaire, observed over time, and then classified into three groups. Tupper et al. suggested that women who abort fall into one of three groups. (1) Women who have inadequate physical and psychological reserves. These women are overly dependent, have difficulty making decisions, become anxious easily, and are ignorant of sex. Tupper et al. viewed the 44 women in this group as intelligent and having insight into their problems. (2) Women who are very intelligent and are socially better adjusted. These 44 women were viewed by the authors as having mixed feelings about the feminine role. They were often pregnant for their husbands' sake. (3) The remaining 12 women were assigned to a "mixed" group for which no general personality characteristics were noted. Tupper et al. concluded that emotional factors seemed to affect the hormonal levels of these women and that psychological support and reassurance seemed to enable some women to preserve the pregnancy.

Tupper and Weil (1962), in a better study, examined 38 habitual aborters over subsequent pregnancies. Nineteen of the women were seen in psychotherapy, whereas 19 were not seen in therapy and served as a control group. The two groups were similar in age, educational level, number of years married, the mean number of previous abortions, and the number of women in each group who had had a child previously. The therapy group had an 84% success rate (full-term live births) but the control group had only a 26% success rate. These results strongly support the contention that supportive counseling or guidance may be an effective intervention for many habitual aborters.

James (1963) discussed the controversy surrounding the treatment of habitual aborters with psychotherapy and the criticism that such "cures" are simply spontaneous; i.e., the chance for successful pregnancy is much higher than realized. He utilized a sample of 781 women to determine the incidence of spontaneous cures in habitual aborters. Of the sample nine women had experienced a trio of consecutive abortions followed by a pregnancy. The outcome of pregnancy for these nine women were six spontaneous abortions and three live births, or an abortion probability of .67. James noted that this probability assumes that these habitual aborters were untreated; however, if any were treated, then this probability is an underestimate. This, however, is a relatively small sample of habitual aborters.

VandenBergh, Taylor, and Drose (1966) approached the question of an underlying emotional conflict in habitual aborters from a different perspective. They studied habitual aborters who had obtained a Shirodkar operation. This operation was devised to correct an apparent weakness of the musculature of the cervix uteri. VandenBergh et al. hypothesized that if a spontaneous abortion is psychologically based, then a Shirodkar operation will produce postpartum psychological problems. Their experimental group consisted of nine habitual aborters; nine women with no history of habitual abortion who had had a successful Shirodkar operation because of an incompetent cervical os served as a control group. The two groups were as closely matched in age and socioeconomic levels as possible.

Of the nine women in the experimental group five underwent a postpartum psychosis. Of the nine women in the control group only one developed a postpartum depression. VandenBergh et al. concluded that in those patients who are forced into motherhood by a Shirodkar operation (i.e., those women in whom abortion appears to have a functional rather than an organic etiology) a postpartum psychosis is likely to occur as the result of exacerbation of underlying emotional conflicts. The authors tempered their conclusions because of two major limitations: (1) the small sample size and (2) the retrospective nature of the study. Another problem with the study is that the Shirodkar operation is designed to prevent fetal wastage due to an incompetent cervical os which usually occurs in the second trimester of pregnancy. This is very likely a different condition from habitual abortion in the first trimester.

Glass and Golbus (1978) reviewed several studies regarding the probability of a habitual aborter's carrying her fourth pregnancy to term. Estimates varied from a 73% risk of abortion in a spontaneous pregnancy preceded by three successive abortions (Malpas, 1938) to only a 24% risk (Warburton & Fraser, 1964). The authors concluded, "There is evidence that some women who have a spontaneous abortion are at somewhat greater risk for a subsequent abortion, but the extent of that risk after three consecutive abortions has not been defined" (p. 258).

Currently only chromosomal abnormalities and uterine malformations have been found to be definitely implicated in the etiology of habitual abortion (Glass & Golbus, 1978). Although assigning an extremely low priority to emotional factors as a cause of habitual abortion, Glass and Golbus recommended psychological support and counseling in the care of couples with habitual abortion.

In summary, it appears most likely that habitual abortion is physiologically or organically based. However, it seems that emotional factors such as stress or trauma may contribute to the difficulties involved in carrying a pregnancy to term. There appears to be little doubt that supportive counseling or psychotherapy is indicated for these women and their husbands. Etiological factors aside, the emotional stress produced by a woman's inability to carry a wanted child to term is severe.

The issue of a personality type or profile of habitual aborters remains unclear. The majority of evidence is clinical, although Grimm's (1962) findings are certainly provocative. The question, of course, is whether these personality factors, if they exist, are part of the etiology or are the result of habitual abortions.

## MEDICALLY NECESSITATED ABORTIONS

Many women obtain abortions for what are described in the literature as "medical reasons." This term typically refers to abortions considered mandatory by a physician to protect the physical health of the women and to abortions considered mandatory because the woman contracted rubella, or other less common infections, while pregnant. Recently, an additional situation has arisen in which an abortion may be viewed as indicated because of the high probability of a genetic disease. Few studies have been conducted to evaluate the psychological effects of a woman's obtaining a "medical abortion"; however, some studies have included an evaluation of reactions to medically necessitated abortions. The results of all these studies have suggested psychological difficulties of a potentially severe magnitude.

Simon, Senturia, and Rothman (1967) conducted a study of 46 abortion patients. Thirty-nine percent (18) were aborted because they contracted rubella, 26% (12) for medical reasons, and 34% for psychiatric reasons. These women were evaluated from 2 months to 10 years following the abortion. They were predominantly white, middle-class, and well educated. Psychiatric disorder was noted in 32 of the 46 women at follow-up. Eleven of the women in the medical group had a psychiatric diagnosis, six being neurotic depression. Five of the 18 women in the rubella group and all 16 women in the psychiatric group were given a psychiatric diagnosis at follow-up.

In reporting on their immediate emotional response to the abortion, the rubella group appeared to have the highest frequency of transient and mild depression whereas the psychiatric group had the lowest frequency of this reaction. In the rubella group 50% were mildly depressed and 12% were markedly depressed; in the medical group the corresponding figures were

25% and 25%; and in the psychiatric group they were 25% and 9%. Positive feelings of relief and well-being were noted by approximately 50% of the women in each group.

Serious psychiatric sequelae were not frequently noted in any of the three groups. In fact, of the six women who had psychiatric hospitalization subsequent to the abortions, only one hospitalization was directly related to the abortion (medical group). The five others were related to chronic psychiatric difficulties, although three were precipitated by subsequent pregnancies and childbirth (rubella group).

Niswander and Patterson (1967) studied 116 women over 16 years of age who had obtained abortions for psychiatric (90), medical (17), or other (9) reasons. Each woman was mailed questionnaires regarding her reactions to the abortion as well as her opinion on its long-term effect on her life. Two-thirds of the women reported feeling better immediately afterward; the figure increased to 82.8% a few weeks after the abortion; and eight months or more following the abortion, 79.3% felt they were emotionally better off. One hundred and ten of the 116 women believed the abortion was the best answer for them. Three women felt negative about the abortion (one woman was aborted for rubella and subsequently had two spontaneous abortions) and three were equivocal (two of these women had medical indications for the abortion).

In further evaluating the women who had mild regret and those who were not sure about their reactions, Niswander and Patterson noted that married gravidas were more likely to have had an unfavorable long-term response than were unmarried patients. Additionally, the reason for the abortion was strongly related to the type of response. Women who had abortions for organic disease were more likely to have an unfavorable reaction immediately than were those aborted for a psychogenic reason.

A study by Peek and Marcus (1966) also compared women obtaining abortions for medical and psychiatric reasons. Each woman was interviewed before the abortion and three to six months after surgery. One-half of the 50 women were aborted because they had contracted rubella during the first trimester of pregnancy. Of these 25 women a psychiatric disorder was noted in 13 but none was a severe disorder. Sixty percent of the nonpsychiatric group wanted the pregnancy but only 4% of the psychiatric group had similar feelings.

This study suggested that only one woman was worse after the abortion. She had been aborted because of rubella, developed a depressive syndrome, improved with psychiatric treatment, and had become pregnant again. Thirty-six percent of the nonpsychiatric group did report mild, brief depressive responses, which had disappeared by the time of follow-up. In line with previous studies only one woman (4%) in the psychiatric group had such a response. Peek and Marcus viewed these mild depressions in the nonpsychiatric group as a mourning reaction since these women wanted the pregnancy but were forced to terminate it because of the possibility of a severely deformed fetus.

Sclare and Geraghty (1971) evaluated 53 women two years after a referral for evaluation for an abortion. Twenty-one patients were aborted for psychiatric reasons, 11 for medical reasons; 21 were denied abortions. These women were comparable with regard to age, marital status, and average number of children. An interview, as well as the Eysenck Personality Inventory (EPI), was utilized in follow-up. The results demonstrated no differences on neuroticism or extroversion across the three groups as measured by the EPI. There were differences with regard to the reactions to the medical decision. With regard to immediate feelings the psychiatric group felt more positive than the medical group, which felt more positive than the group denied abortion. Two years after the abortion a shift in acceptance level was noted in the reaction of the medical group. The acceptance level, or number of women reporting agreement with the medical decision, dropped from nine to five over the two-year period following the abortion. This change was apparently determined by the positive wishes of these women in regard to the pregnancy and their disappointment and negative feelings with regard to the loss of a wanted child.

In 1975 Blumberg, Golbus, and Hanson published a paper on the psychological reactions in couples who had obtained abortions for genetic indications. Thirteen couples electing abortion following amniocentesis for prenatal detection of genetic defect were studied. (The MMPI and a questionnaire were mailed to 15 couples; however, only 13 interviews were successfully arranged so only these couples were included.)

The MMPI profiles of the women were very close to the population mean profile; however, the profiles of the men showed some elevations in the scales of depression, hysteria, sociopathy, femininity, and hypomania. The elevation on femininity was seen as the result of the generally high educational levels of these men. The elevations on hysteria and depression were noted to be common in individuals experiencing underlying tension or anxiety.

In spite of the lack of findings with regard to depression on the MMPI profiles of the women, interview data suggested that depression was a very frequent response immediately following abortion. Only 2 of 13 women and 4 of 11 men failed to mention depression in describing their emotional reaction to the abortion. Since three of these six people had MMPI profiles that suggested a tendency to deny emotional problems, the authors proposed that the actual incidence of depression might have been as high as 92% among the women and 82% among the men in this small sample. Although the intensity and duration of the depressive reaction described varied with the subjects, Blumberg et al. concluded that these reactions were more severe than those described in the literature for women having abortions for psychosocial reasons.

Despite the small sample and limited measurements used, the study by Blumberg et al. did not appear to show reactions significantly different from reactions to elective, psychiatric, and other types of medical abortions. The 13 families experienced emotional and interpersonal difficulties so severe that 4 couples separated following the abortion. Several factors appear to have been involved. These pregnancies were all wanted and the pregnancies were all terminated in the second trimester, after quickening had occurred.

Quickening makes the issue of how women think about the fetus very important. Senay (1970) described an inhibition of the normal fantasy process in women requesting early elective or therapeutic abortions. This inhibition consists of the woman's not developing fantasies about the fetus she is carrying. These women do not daydream about the sex of the child or its physical appearance and, in fact, reported no fantasy material about the fetus. This is unusual as most women have many fantasies, daydreams, etc., about the unborn child. Wallerstein, Kurtz, and Bar-Din (1972) presented some cases that suggested that a woman's fantasies about the fetus may serve as guides to the type of reaction she might have to an abortion. The fantasy content, as well as the frequency and intensity of the fantasies, is important. For example, a woman who imagines that she is murdering her baby when she obtains an abortion is likely to remain preoccupied and distressed about the abortion for many months. On the other hand, a woman who has inhibited or repressed fantasies regarding the fetus is less likely to experience conflict and remain preoccupied with the abortion. A woman who is happy about her pregnancy is likely to have positive fantasies about her baby and is likely to react with sorrow or grief if the pregnancy is terminated. All of the women in the Blumberg et al. (1975) study had decided to abort a wanted child about whom they had positive fantasies; therefore, the probability of an adverse reaction was increased.

Although there are few available data, the study by Blumberg et al. (1975) suggested that women who obtain abortions for genetic reasons following amniocentesis may be at risk for severe psychological reactions. These women have to deal with several factors that increase the likelihood of depression and lowered self-worth. In addition to dealing with the loss of a desired pregnancy, the woman may have already begun to think of the fetus as a separate person and thus she must face the loss on a more intensely emotional level. Additionally, the presence of the genetic problem may serve to increase feelings of inadequacy or failure in one or both partners. At least one member of each couple had to face the possibility of the stigma and guilt of being a carrier of a genetic disease and had to face the fact that they had failed to produce a healthy child. For many this inability or failure produced serious psychological sequelae and resulted in serious disruptions in their family lives.

One difficulty with the medical literature dealing with the psychological or psychiatric responses to medical abortions is highlighted by Babikian (1976). He describes that a review of 200 papers on abortion revealed that "each author had an emotional committment either to the protagonist or the antagonist camp" (p. 1497). Thus it is very likely that the confusing and contradictory literature describing either significant psychiatric sequelae, or no psychiatric sequelae, may be due to observer bias. He further comments from his review of the literature that psychiatric illness present before pregnancy, for which the abortion was performed, showed no significant improvement after abortion. And, these women with psychiatric illness antedating pregnancy had more difficulty in dealing successfully with abortion than did the psychiatrically healthier group.

It seems likely that there are two groups of women to be found in the population obtaining abortions primarily for psychiatric indications. The first group is probably the smaller and contains those women who have significant or severe psychiatric illness preexisting the pregnancy. The second and probably larger group, particularly as abortion laws have been liberalized, includes those women without demonstrable psychiatric illness prior to the pregnancy but for whom the pregnancy represents enough of a psychological or social stress that they seek abortions in order to prevent the development of manifest psychiatric illness. It is unlikely in the former group that an abortion will significantly improve psychiatric symptomatology or functioning after the abortion. Such abortions may be performed because of health professionals' fears that the chronically psychiatrically ill mother will be unable to care for the child. In these women with compromised psychological functioning the stress of the pregnancy and the abortion may at least transiently make things considerably worse. However, for the second group the abortion may indeed reduce stress, improve psychiatric symptomatology which developed acutely during the pregnancy because of the pregnancy, and be more likely to be viewed as a positive procedure in the months that follow the abortion.

In summary, it appears that women who obtain abortions for nonpsychiatric medical reasons are the most likely to experience problems regarding the decision. These women have desired the pregnancy and usually have begun actively to fantasize about the behavior and characteristics of the unborn child. The decision to abort because of the mother's medical problems or exposure to rubella appears to produce conflict and stress, which may be reduced by the abortion itself. Following the abortion a short-term depressive reaction occurs in one-third to one-half of these women and suggests the need for support to the woman and her husband at this point in time. Less frequently, more long-term difficulties occur in terms of depressive states. A likely hypothesis is that women who find themselves unable to have another child remain conflicted, whereas those who are able to fulfill this desire at some point in the future are able to obtain closure on the experience. Those women who have abortions for genetic considerations appear to be at extremely high risk for personal psychological difficulties, as well as for family discord and disruption. Because of the possibility of such emotional difficulties, as well as the complexity of the decision to abort in this situation; counseling of these couples around the time of the abortion decision and several months afterward would appear to be of primary importance.

## THERAPEUTIC ABORTIONS

One of the earliest and most frequently cited studies concerning a woman's reaction to a therapeutic abortion was conducted in Sweden by Ekblad (1955). In evaluating the postabortion functioning of 54 women he noted several relationships that subsequent research has supported. For example, he noted that women who were coerced into an abortion had more psychological difficulties following the abortion. Additionally, he found that those women who were considered abnormal or as having a psychiatric disturbance before the abortion were the most likely to have psychiatric difficulties following the abortion. In spite of reporting feelings of guilt and self-reproach the majority of women (90%) functioned well and had no reduction in work capacity.

The studies that have followed have employed a variety of procedures and outcome measures to evaluate the psychological reactions of women to therapeutic abortion; however, the majority of studies have supported Ekblad findings.

A commonly employed methodology is to contact a group of women several months or years following an abortion and evaluate their current status as well as feelings about the abortion. Niswander and Patterson (1967) utilized questionnaires, as did Todd (1972), Ewing and Rouse (1973), and Whittington (1970). The studies found that the majority of women adjusted very well emotionally following abortion.

Niswander and Patterson (1967) obtained an 87.9% return rate on questionnaires sent to 132 women who had obtained therapeutic abortions one to three years previously. Two-thirds of these women reported feeling better immediately following the abortion. The percentage of women who felt better rose to 82% eight months later. Only five women sampled regretted having obtained the abortion.

Todd (1972) contacted patients one to three years postabortion. He obtained replies from 78 of 83 women, 4 of whom had not obtained an abortion in spite of recommendations. Ninety-one percent reported no adverse sequelae from the abortion. Only one woman appeared to be having adverse sequelae directly related to the abortion and she had been chronically depressed. Todd also obtained data concerning subsequent pregnancies and found that seven women had become pregnant again.

Ewing and Rouse (1973) sent questionnaires two weeks to two years postabortion to 300 women. Replies were obtained from 126 women who had obtained abortions on psychiatric grounds. Fifty-two of these women had a history of psychiatric illness prior to the pregnancy. The women with a history of psychiatric illness as well as the women who had a recent onset of psychiatric illness reported that their general (100% and 96%, respectively) and emotional (96% and 92%) health was better or normal postabortion. The only significant difference between the two groups was that insomnia was more frequent in those women with a psychiatric history. Ewing and Rouse commented that if the abortion procedure is carried out under good medical and legal conditions at the request of the woman herself, unfavorable emotional reactions are unlikely even in women with previous psychiatric problems.

Whittington (1970) sent letters to 196 women who had requested a therapeutic abortion during nine months in 1967. Of these women 134 had obtained a therapeutic abortion; 62 had been denied the abortion. Although some of these abortions were obtained because the fetus was determined to be defective, and some because of the mother's physical health (frequency not reported), the majority were performed because of the belief that the women would develop serious psychiatric problems if she had the baby. Many of the women appeared to have moved as letters were returned unopened, and many women were not willing to participate. A total of 31 of the 134 women obtaining abortions completed the questionnaire. Sixty-eight percent reported that their mental health was better, 19% reported it was probably better, 10% reported it might be better, and 3% reported it was probably worse as a result of the abortion. Nine of the 31 women had experienced emotional symptoms since the abortion and 8 of the 9 had seen a mental health professional.

Levene and Rigney (1970) conducted a retrospective study of 70 women granted therapeutic abortions. The women responded to questionnaires three to five months postabortion. Each patient was asked to complete the following: an 18-item depression rating scale comparing their current feelings with their immediate postabortion feelings, a multiple affect adjective checklist regarding their present mood only, and a questionnaire concerning their postabortion psychiatric help, whether they would have the abortion again, and how they felt about the procedure.

Eighty percent (46) of the women participated in the study. Depression, as measured by the depression checklist, was significantly lower following the abortion. Eight patients who reported increased depression did *not* believe it was related to the abortion. The average scores obtained on the adjective checklist concerning present feelings were no different from the average scores of female college students. The majority of women had a positive attitude toward the abortion, and 38 would have the abortion again.

These studies, utilizing different types of self-report measures, suggest that the majority of women who obtained therapeutic abortions for *psychiatric* reasons believed that their mental health had improved since obtaining the abortion. Equally as important, only a very small percentage of women in each study reported increased emotional difficulties since the abortion.

Another type of retrospective approach utilized in abortion research involves more direct but perhaps less objective contact with a woman several months or years after her abortion. Some studies report data obtained in semistructured interviews and others combine data from psychological tests with interview data to describe postabortion level of functioning.

Simon, Senturia, and Rothman (1967) were able to obtain interviews and test data from 46 women, 16 of whom had obtained abortions for psychiatric reasons 2 to 10 years previously. Eight of these 16 women reported positive responses and feelings of relief. Mild depression was reported by four of the women and one reported marked depression. No immediate emotional response could be determined from the data of the remaining three. Simon et al. also evaluated the amount of conscious guilt felt by the women in the study. Four of the women in the psychiatric group reported marked conscious guilt relating to the abortion. These women reported a diminution of guilt feelings as time progressed. Some information regarding the subsequent level of functioning of the women in the psychiatric group was obtained. For example, 2 of the 16 women required hospitalization; however, both of these hospitalizations were precipitated by events other than the abortion and appeared to be part of preexisting psychiatric problems. Three other women developed depressive reactions of moderate severity in which the abortion was a factor. None of these women required hospitalization.

Simon et al. concluded that these results suggest that women who obtain abortions for psychiatric reasons will not necessarily become more disturbed. On the contrary, the abortion may serve as a stabilizing factor or may be considered insignificant. With certain types of psychopathology there may be an increased incidence of mild depression immediately following the abortion. Finally, serious psychiatric illness following an abortion is only rarely precipitated by, or related to, the abortion. Subsequent problems are typically related to preexisting psychological problems.

Patt, Rappaport, and Barglow (1969) followed up 32 women who obtained therapeutic abortions during the previous four years. Interviews with 26 women were conducted; 5 women were not interviewed but their psychiatrists were; and 1 woman refused to participate. For 20 of the 35 women prompt remission of psychiatric symptoms occurred. Of the remaining 15 women, 50% exhibited symptoms (self-multilation, promiscuity, or depression) that related to preexisting problems. The other 50% developed symptoms in response to the abortion. Two women who attempted suicide in response to the abortion stated that the abortion had been performed against their will. Perhaps the most important finding was that 13 of these 15 women stated that the abortion was the best alternative for them in spite of not thereby obtaining any relief from psychiatric symptoms. They believed that their problems would be worse if they had not had the abortion.

Pare and Raven (1970) compared 128 women who had been recommended for and obtained a therapeutic abortion to 120 patients who had been refused an abortion. In the terminated group all but two women were glad that the pregnancy had been terminated. Both of these women had not wanted the abortion but had obtained it because of pressure by their husbands. Although mild feelings of guilt or loss were not unusual, they typically lasted only one or two weeks. Only 17 cases (13%) lasted for longer than three months. There was a striking lack of serious psychiatric sequelae in this group of women.

Several studies have attempted to evaluate women preabortion and postabortion in order to assess psychological changes that might occur or problems that might develop.

Brody, Meikle, and Gerritse (1971) evaluated 177 women applying for a therapeutic abortion and compared them to 58 controls (women in the same state of pregnancy). Of the 117, 94 were granted abortions; 52 of these women had tubal ligations. Several tests were utilized as dependent measures and were administered to the experimental group when the abortion was requested. Repeat testing was six weeks postabortion, six months postabortion, and one year post abortion. For the controls and for the women whose request was rejected, readministration took place six weeks after the expected term date. The results of the testing demonstrated that the applicants for abortion reported a marked degree of psychological disturbance on the MMPI; the scores of the control group fell in the normal range.

Significant changes on the MMPI were noted as early as six weeks postabortion on every scale except Scale 5 (M–F). Compared to preabortion levels a downward trend in pathology, as measured by the MMPI, was noted for all women at the one year follow-up. Those women who had been denied an abortion showed no change on the clinical scales eight to nine months later; however, the number of women who were willing to participate was so small that no valid conclusions could be made. Brody et al. concluded that there is no support for a guilt reaction postabortion. On the contrary, the women in their study showed psychological improvement postabortion.

Margolis, Davison, Hanson, Loos, and Mikkelsen (1971) evaluated 50 women seeking abortions for psychiatric (44) and medical (6) reasons. A questionnaire, the MMPI, a psychiatric evaluation, and an interview by a social worker were obtained preabortion. Follow-up data were obtained for 43 women three to six months following the abortion. The test results following the abortion were more frequently in the normal range. The follow-up interviews showed corresponding positive changes in that 29 patients reported positive changes. Only 4 women had negative reactions such as guilt or fear of men and 10 women indicated no change. Margolis et al.

interpreted these findings to suggest that terminations of pregnancy do not aggravate mental illness; rather, they often benefit the patient by improving her life situation.

Niswander, Singer, and Singer (1972) evaluated 65 abortion patients and 20 maternity patients shortly before their respective medical events. The MMPI was administered to all women and the scores were then rated on a scale of one to five by a clinical psychologist for four dimensions: overall adjustment, depression, anxiety, and impulsivity. The psychologist did not know in which group any women belonged. The results indicated that the abortion group as compared to the maternity patients had significantly higher ratings on all four dimensions, but the greatest difference was on impulsivity. Postoperative scores were less discrepant; however, significant differences between the two groups were found for anxiety and impulsivity. The authors interpreted the significant decrease in the scores of the abortion group as reflecting the reduction in stress that accompanied the abortion.

Ford, Castelnuovo-Tedesco, and Long (1971) evaluated 30 women preabortion and postabortion. These abortions were requested on mental health grounds. During the preabortion interview the women reported depression, anxiety, insomnia, and headaches. During the postabortion interview most women reported improvement (43%, marked improvement; 62%, moderate symptom relief). Only three stated that they were more upset postabortion. The authors also noted that the more normal patients benefited most from an abortion whereas the more disturbed women tended to incorporate it into their illness.

Jacobs, Garcia, Rickels, and Prencil (1974) evaluated 57 women prior to abortion using a preabortion questionnaire, the MMPI, the Patient Symptom Check List (64-item checklist of common psychoneurotic complaints), the Zung Self-rating Depression Scale (20-item scale of depressive complaints), and the Clyde Mood Scale (48-item checklist yielding six factors: friendly, aggressive, clear-thinking, sleepy, unhappy, and dizzy). Forty-three women were contacted four weeks postabortion. The Symptom Check List, Self-rating Depression Scale, and Clyde Mood Scale were readministered at that time and each woman completed a postabortion questionnaire as well. The women in this study were granted abortions if it was believed that the woman's physical, mental, or social well-being might be impaired by continuing the pregnancy.

Following the abortion a significant reduction in distress occurred on the Symptom Check List and the Self-rating Depression Scale total scores, in all but one of the Symptom Check List factors, and in three of six Clyde Mood Scale factors. Symptom reduction was particularly marked on items that are commonly experienced during pregnancy, i.e., physiological items. A subjective report by women confirmed these data. Sixty percent of the patients were feeling better, 28% the same, and only 12% felt worse.

Sclare and Geraghty (1971) compared three groups of women: patients accepted for abortions on psychiatric grounds; patients denied abortions on psychiatric grounds; and patients accepted for abortions on medical grounds. The women were interviewed at the time of applying for the abortion; two years later they were given a semistructured interview and the Eysenck Personality Inventory. There were no significant changes on the extroversion or neuroticism factors during the two evaluations nor were there significant differences between groups. Both abortion groups were happier or reported better subsequent mental health than did the group refused abortion.

In summary, it appears that abortion is often beneficial to the woman experiencing psychiatric problems who seeks to have the abortion. The apparent reduction of stress following a therapeutic abortion has been noted by many authors as contributing to improved mental health in most women obtaining abortions of this type. Direct measures such as self-report questionnaires concerning level of functioning since the abortion, changes in affect, and somatic complaints also suggest decreased somatic symptoms and decreases in depression following abortions obtained for psychiatric reasons. The MMPI, an objective but indirect measure, also supports the theory that the woman who obtains an abortion for psychiatric reasons will exhibit less pathology after the abortion.

The reaction of each individual is impossible to predict; however, the studies reviewed suggest that the less severe the psychiatric disturbance the higher the level of functioning following the abortion. Several authors have noted that women with severe and chronic psychiatric problems often appear to incorporate the abortion into their psychopathology. That is, a woman who has a documented delusional system in which she feels victimized or persecuted may expand this system to include the abortion, which she may subsequently believe was forced upon her. It should be noted, however, that the denial of abortion to this type of woman may result in just as many pathological distortions in addition to adding the realistic stress of a child for whom she must care. Thus, it appears that an abortion may be the best alternative in a problematic situation. A woman whose history suggests the possibility of such a reaction needs intervention by a mental health professional during the abortion crisis and in the subsequent years.

## FACTORS AFFECTING A WOMAN'S PSYCHOLOGICAL RESPONSE TO AN ABORTION

In the preceding sections we discussed many of the different types of abortions, as well as the research regarding the outcome of each type of abortion. For the most part, a large majority of women do not have psychiatric sequelae to abortions performed for psychiatric reasons nor do they have psychiatric sequelae following spontaneous and/or habitual abortions. Women who obtain abortions for medical reasons have a higher probability of having psychological difficulties following the abortion; however, the vast majority of women do not have long-term psychiatric problems following abortion. Thus, in a large sample of women having abortions, one would predict that few women would have severe psychiatric sequelae or become so disturbed that hospitalization would be required. Nonetheless, for the person concerned with the particular reaction or subsequent mental health of a specific woman, it is important to understand the factors that may adversely affect her. That is, although from a research point of view we can say that a woman is unlikely to have an adverse reaction, from a clinical point of view it becomes important to look at the various factors that are influencing an individual woman so that we may be able to predict with some degree of accuracy her unique reaction to the abortion.

In this section, we will focus attention on some variables that may warn of greater potential for negative psychological consequences for a particular woman. A variety of potential indicators of psychological distress following an abortion have been suggested. Although the majority of studies have involved women who have obtained elective abortions, the results clearly suggest factors affecting all types of abortions.

The work of Adler (1975) has suggested a theoretical framework within which we can evaluate a given woman's potential reaction to an abortion.

Adler (1975) attempted to classify the various types of emotional response to an abortion. She obtained ratings on the following emotions postabortion: embarrassment, regret, guilt, relief, anxiety, shame, fear of disapproval, anger, happiness, depression, doubt, and disappointment in self. A factor analysis of the ratings of these emotions led to two important findings. First, emotional responses did not fall along a simple positive-negative dimension; rather, a woman may feel both positive emotions such as happiness and relief while at the same time experiencing the negative emotions of guilt and regret. Second, Adler found that the negative emotions formed two separate factors: one that appears related to socially based norms and another that appears related to personal, or internally based, responses. This suggests that two different sources may produce negative emotions or difficulties for women. Shame, guilt, and fear of disapproval are examples of reactions to norm violations, whereas regret, depression, and doubt seem to be based on the meaning of the pregnancy and the abortion for the individual woman.

Thus, the results of Adler's study suggest that the negative emotional reactions of an individual woman to an abortion are produced by two distinct sets of forces. The woman's social environment—the attitudes and beliefs of the culture in which she lives—will determine the extent of social disapproval or socially based negative emotions she experiences. A second set of forces arises from the woman's internal world: the personal reactions she has to the pregnancy and the resulting negative emotions she may feel as a result of the loss of the pregnancy. Finally, Adler noted that relief and happiness, positive emotions, were a separate and more powerful factor in her study. Adler suggested that the strongest emotional reaction a woman may have will be relief and happiness; however, these two emotions are unrelated to the factors that influence the intensity of the negative emotions. With regard to the personal variables that may influence a woman's reaction to an abortion, age has been cited in several studies as an important factor (Lash, 1975; Payne et al., 1976). The most frequent finding is that young women are more likely to experience difficulty following an abortion than are older women. Adler (1975) found age to be a significant variable that was inversely related to the intensity of negative emotions; that is, the younger the woman the more likely she was to experience the socially based as well as the internally based negative emotions. Margolis et al. (1971), Wallerstein, Kurtz, and Bar-Din (1972), and Perez-Reyes and Falk (1973) all noted clinical examples of adolescent girls who had a particularly difficult time postabortion. These authors all suggested that the developmental stage of adolescence, as well as the influence of other factors such as the family's reaction, put the young adolescent girl at high risk for psychological difficulties following an abortion.

Another factor that appears to influence a woman's reaction to an abortion is her plan to have children in the future. Not unexpectedly, the available research suggests that women who before the abortion had planned to bear children are likely to experience more health concerns, mood fluctuations, and somatic complaints than are women who did not want to have or who were ambivalent about having children (Greenglass, 1977).

Payne, Kravitz, Notman, and Anderson (1976) suggested that a woman's religious beliefs may also affect her reaction to an abortion. These authors noted that Catholicism was associated with depression and shame following abortion. Adler's (1975) findings do not support this notion; however, there appears to have been a self-selection factor in the Adler study in that Catholic women were the least likely to participate in the follow-up portion of the study. On the other hand, Adler did note some significant findings with regard to religiosity. These findings suggested that religiosity as reflected in church attendance did show a significant relationship with socially based negative emotions. That is, women who attended church frequently (once a month or more) were likely to experience socially based negative emotions more frequently than were women who did not attend church.

Using a more global approach, the studies of Belsey, Greer, Lal, Lewis, and Beard (1977), Lash (1975), and Payne, Kravitz, Notman, and Anderson (1976) all suggested that those women whose overall adjustment, both personal and social, appears to be good preabortion will have the least difficulty postabortion. That is, in general, preabortion levels of functioning appear to be the most reliable indicator of postabortion levels of functioning. Women who have no psychiatric problems are least likely to have a psychiatric disturbance postabortion. On the other hand, women whose social history reflects difficulty in getting along with peers, getting along with family, and adjusting to school or work are most likely to have difficulties with regard to socially based negative emotions.

Another approach to attempting to predict a woman's postabortion level of functioning has been taken by several authors who have examined the decisionmaking process regarding an abortion. Studies by Ford et al. (1971) and by Niswander and Patterson (1967) noted that postabortion difficulties in women whose families did not support the abortion decision were severe. These findings led Bracken, Phil, Hachamovitch, and Grossman (1974) to hypothesize that reactions to abortion may be strongly influenced by the reactions of significant others in the woman's life. They hypothesized that a high-quality decision, that is, one that had been thought about at length and discussed with important others, would be associated with more positive responses to an abortion than would a low-quality decision. They argued further that the social milieu, as well as the support of important others, was critical to the reaction of a woman obtaining an abortion.

The findings of Bracken et al. (1974) support this hypothesis. They also found that for the older married woman or the older single woman, the knowledge and support of her husband and/or partner was the most critical factor. If the husband or partner was aware of the abortion and supportive of it, the woman was more likely to have a positive reaction. For the younger single woman it was more critical for her parents to be aware of and support the decision than for her partner to do so. Disapproval or a lack of support from a family was highly correlated with emotional distress following an abortion.

Finally, it is important for a woman obtaining an abortion to come to a relatively firm decision concerning the abortion. The woman who remains ambivalent regarding the abortion is the most likely to experience psychological distress and emotional disturbance following the abortion. Postabortion difficulties noted in women who felt ambivalent about an abortion or felt coerced into it were noted in studies by Smith (1973), Belsey et al. (1977), Lash (1975), and Payne et al. (1976).

To summarize, the social environment in which the woman functions, as well as her personal needs and desires with regard to pregnancy, are major factors affecting the intensity of negative emotions she may experience following an abortion. The older woman with no history of emotional difficulties and whose husband favors and supports the abortion is most likely to experience no emotional distress or difficulties following an abortion.

On the other hand, young single women who are not involved in a stable relationship or whose parents are opposed to the abortion are at risk for symptomatic responses. These factors, as well as the decisionmaking process itself, can be critical. Those women who carefully think through the decision concerning an abortion are unlikely to have severe psychiatric or psychological sequelae following an abortion. On the other hand, those women who feel coerced into an abortion or who continue to be ambivalent about obtaining an abortion are very likely to have psychological problems following an abortion. We should note that although most of these studies investigated elective abortions, the results clearly suggest factors affecting all types of abortions.

## RECOMMENDATIONS

The literature on elective (or birth control) abortions, as well as the literature on therapeutic abortions, i.e., those obtained for psychiatric reasons in a relatively healthy population, suggests that the modal response to the abortion may be one of transient depressive mood with the distinct possibility that positive emotions will predominate (Calhoun, Selby, & King, 1976). Our conclusions suggest strongly that these findings on elective and therapeutic abortions are for the most part not applicable to abortions undertaken for medical or genetic reasons. It is important, then, to the professional who performs abortion counseling to be aware of the conditions that produce the request for abortion.

In general, the reactions to spontaneous and habitual abortions are similar in that they both appear to involve grief reactions to the loss of a planned and wanted child. For the woman who has experienced a spontaneous abortion, crisis counseling for her and her husband appears to be indicated. Therapeutic intervention to facilitate the grieving process has been found to be of benefit in such cases and we recommend it.

For the couple obtaining a medical abortion for genetic reasons or because of some defect of the fetus, thorough preparation for the procedure as well as follow-up for several months thereafter is indicated. Specifically, for the couple obtaining an abortion for genetic reasons, there are several critical issues, in addition to the loss of the child, with which they must deal. The inability to produce a normal child may be a severe blow to the self-esteem of the partner who is the carrier. This loss of self-esteem may in turn result in severe depression, which may affect the marriage of the couple involved. In view of the complexity of the issues for the genetic carrier as well as the resulting disruption in the marital relationship, more intensive intervention involving preparation for the abortion, grieving over the loss, and resolution of the issue of future pregnancies is mandatory.

Mental health professionals who assist women in deciding about abortions and those who assist women postabortion should be aware of the importance of the decision to abort in postabortion levels of functioning. The woman who is ambivalent about the abortion or whose social support system (family, friends, religious group, etc.) is opposed to the abortion will require more extensive and intensive support following the abortion. We think it desirable for patients who are ambivalent or who have social support systems that do not agree with the decision to abort to have routine contact with a social worker, psychologist, or individual with similar training after the abortion occurs.

We also suggest that women who have characteristics that we have identified as potential indicators of psychological distress postabortion be followed on a routine basis. This at risk population would include women who are young, single, have a religion opposed to abortion, attend church more frequently than once a month, and who plan to have children at some point in the future. Professional assistance for these women should be readily available, and follow-up sessions should be encouraged for the woman who experiences distress postabortion.

Group counseling appears to be quite effective specifically with women whose difficulty around the abortion has to do with internally based negative emotions. Thus, group counseling would be of greatest benefit to married women who are older and who have decided to have an abortion with the support and encouragement of the husband or partner. These women appear to be able to benefit most from a group setting and do not have to be seriously concerned with being socially rejected. Abortion patients who are young, single, and lack the support of family and friends would seem to be the least appropriate candidates for group therapy regarding responses to abortion. Rather, these women and adolescents would benefit most from individual counseling.

Professionals who routinely provide abortion counseling, both preabortion and postabortion, might benefit from psychological support themselves. One factor that may increase the probability of burnout in counselors is constant exposure to situations in which the abortion is difficult. Thus, those counselors who work in a hospital or clinic setting in which they must constantly deal not only with the woman who is requesting the abortion but also with the medical personnel who perform this procedure will be the most highly stressed. Performing abortions has been documented to be highly stressful work, especially as the issue of when the fetus becomes a separate individual must be faced on a personal level by each of the professional staff. It would appear mandatory for abortion counselors functioning in this type of setting to receive psychological support and supervision from other mental health professionals on a routine basis. Those people who are providing abortion counseling in settings quite distant from the setting in which the abortion is performed may be less susceptible to burnout and may need less support from other professionals.

Because abortion has often been regarded as a crisis, many professionals expect all abortion patients to experience psychological difficulties. Data, however, seem actually to suggest the opposite: women who undergo abortion may actually experience a predominance of positive emotions (Calhoun, Selby, & King, 1976). When the abortion is necessitated by medical reasons (health threat to the mother or defect in the fetus) or grave psychiatric problems (severe and chronic mental illness of the mother), positive emotions may not be as predominant as with elective abortions or abortions performed for psychiatric reasons in which the mental health of the mother is not chronically impaired. Nevertheless, while on the one hand we are recommending routine psychological follow-up of abortion patients with certain characteristics and patients obtaining certain types of abortions, we also caution professionals not to produce iatrogenic psychological distress in abortion patients simply because they as professionals view abortion as a crisis. Abortion does seem to be a crisis of lesser or greater magnitude for many patients. For many, however, abortion may not be a crisis at all.

## REFERENCES

Abernathy, V. The abortion constellation: early history and present relationships. *Archives of General Psychiatry,* 1973, *29,* 346–350.

Addelson, F. Induced abortion: source of guilt or growth? *American Journal of Orthopsychiatry,* 1973, *43,* 815–823.

Adler, N. E. Emotional responses of women following therapeutic abortion. *American Journal of Orthopsychiatry,* 1975, *45,* 446–454.

Aron, P., and Amark, C. Prognosis when abortion granted but not carried out. *Acta Psychiatrica Scandinavica,* 1961, *36,* 203–278.

Athanasiou, R., Oppel, W., Michelson, L., Unger, T., and Yager, M. Psychiatric sequelae to term birth and induced early and late abortion: a longitudinal study. *Family Planning Perspectives,* 1973, *5,* 227–231.

Babikan, H. M. Abortion. In A. N. Freedman, H. I. Kaplan & D. J. Sadock (Eds.), Comprehensive Textbook of Psychiatry (Vol. 2). Baltimore: Williams & Wilkins Co., 1976.

Baudry, F., and Wiener, A. The pregnant patient in conflict about abortion: a challenge for the obstetrician. *American Journal of Obstetrics and Gynecology,* 1974, *119,* 705–711.

Belsey, E. M., Greer, H. S., Lal, S., Lewis, S. C., and Beard, R. W. Predictive factors in emotional response to abortion: King's termination study. *Social Science and Medicine,* 1977, *11,* 71–82.

Blumberg, B. D., Golbus, M. S., and Hanson, K. H. The psychological sequelae of abortion performed for a genetic indication. *American Journal of Obstetrics and Gynecology,* 1975, *122,* 799–808.

Blumenfield, M. Psychological factors involved in request for elective abortion. *Journal of Clinical Psychiatry,* 1978, *39,* 17–25.

Bolter, S. The psychiatrist's role in therapeutic abortion: the unwilling accomplice. *American Journal of Psychiatry,* 1962, *119,* 312–316.

Bracken, M. B., Phil, M., Hachamovitch, M., and Grossman, G. The decision to abort and psychological sequelae. *Journal of Nervous and Mental Disease,* 1974, *158,* 154–162.

Brekke, B. *Abortion in the United States.* New York: Harper, 1958.

BREWER, C. Incidence of post-abortion psychosis. *Obstetrical and Gynecological Survey,* 1977, *32,* 600–601.

BRODY, H., MEIKLE, S., and GERRITSE, R. Therapeutic abortion: a prospective study. *American Journal of Obstetrics and Gynecology,* 1971, *109,* 347–353.

CALHOUN, L. G., SELBY, J. W., and KING, H. E. *Dealing with crisis.* Englewood Cliffs: Prentice-Hall, 1976.

CASADY, M. Abortion: no lasting emotional scars. *Psychology Today,* 1974, *8,* 148–149.

CONNELL, E. B. Abortion patterns, techniques, and results. *Fertility and Sterility,* 1973, *24,* 78–91.

CORNEY, R. T., and HORTON, F. T. Pathological grief following spontaneous abortion. *American Journal of Psychiatry,* 1974, *131,* 825–827.

CVEJIC, H., LIPPER, I., KINEK, R. A., and BEUGANIN, P. Follow-up of 50 adolescent girls two years after abortion. *Canadian Medical Association Journal,* 1977, *116,* 44–46.

DYCHE, M. E. Grief work after a miscarriage. *Maternal-Child Nursing Journal,* 1973, *1,* 281–288.

EDITORIAL. psychological sequelae of therapeutic abortion. *British Medical Journal,* 1976, *1,* 1239.

EKBLAD, M. Induced abortion on psychiatric grounds. *Acta Psychiatrica Scandinavica,* 1955, *31* (supplement 99), 1–238.

EVANS, D. A., and GUSDON, J. P., JR. Postabortion attitudes. *North Carolina Medical Journal,* 1973, *34,* 271–273.

EWING, J., and ROUSE, B. Therapeutic abortion and a prior psychiatric history. *American Journal of Psychiatry,* 1973, *130,* 37–40.

FLECK, S. Some psychiatric aspects of abortion. *Journal of Nervous and Mental Disease,* 1970, *151,* 42–50.

FINGERER, M. E. Psychological sequelae of abortion: anxiety and depression. *Journal of Community Psychology,* 1973, *1,* 221–225.

FORSSMAN, H., and THUIVE, I. One hundred and twenty children born after application for therapeutic abortion refused. *Acta Psychiatrica Scandinavica,* 1966, *42,* 71–88.

FORD, C. V., CASTELNUOVO-TEDESCO, P., and LONG, K. Abortion: is it a therapeutic procedure in psychiatry? *Journal of the American Medical Association,* 1971, *218,* 1173–1178.

———. Women who seek therapeutic abortion: a comparison with women who complete their pregnancies. *American Journal of Psychiatry,* 1972, *129,* 546–552.

FREUNDT, L. Surveys in induced spontaneous abortions in the Copenhagen area. *Acta Psychiatrica Scandinavica,* 1964, *40* (supplement 80), 235–237.

FRIEDMAN, C. M. Making abortion consultation therapeutic. *American Journal of Psychiatry,* 1973, *130,* 1257–1261.

FRIEDMAN, C. M., GREENSPAN, R., and MITTLEMAN, F. The decision making process and the outcome of therapeutic abortion. *American Journal of Psychiatry,* 1974, *131,* 1332–1337.

GLASS, R. H., and GOLBUS, M. S., Habitual abortion. *Fertility and Sterility,* 1978, *29,* 257–265.

GREENGLASS, E. R. Therapeutic abortion, fertility plans, and psychological sequelae. *American Journal of Orthopsychiatry,* 1977, *47,* 119–126.

GRIMM, E. R. Psychological investigation of habitual abortion. *Psychosomatic Medicine,* 1962, *24,* 369–378.

HAMILL, E., AND INGRAM, T. M. Psychiatric and social factors in the abortion decision. *British Medical Journal,* 1974, *1,* 229–232.

HARDIN, G. Abortion versus the right to life: the evil of mandatory motherhood. *Psychology Today,* 1974, *8,* 42–50.

Hathaway, S. R., and Briggs, P. F. Some normative data on new MMPI scales. *Journal of Clinical Psychology,* 1957, *13,* 364–368.

Jacobs, D., Garcia, C. R., Rickels, K., and Prencil, J. A prospective study on the psychological effects of therapeutic abortion. *Comprehensive Psychiatry,* 1974, *15,* 523–534.

James, W. H. The problem of spontaneous abortion: the efficacy of psychotherapy. *American Journal of Obstetrics and Gynecology,* 1963, *85,* 38–40.

Javert, C. T. Stress and habitual abortion. *Obstetrics and Gynecology,* 1954, *3,* 298–301.

Kaij, L., Malmquist, A., and Nilsson, A. Psychiatric aspects of spontaneous abortion. Part 2: The importance of bereavement, attachment, and neurosis in early life. *Journal of Psychosomatic Research,* 1969, *13,* 53–59.

Kane, F. J., Jr., and Lachenbruch, P. A. Adolescent pregnancy: a study of aborters and non-aborters. *American Journal of Orthopsychiatry,* 1973, *43,* 796–803.

Kummer, J. M. Post-abortion psychiatric illness: a myth? *American Journal of Psychiatry,* 1963, *119,* 980–983.

Lash, B. Short-term psychiatric sequelae to therapeutic termination of pregnancy. *British Journal of Psychiatry,* 1975, *126,* 173–177.

Lebensohn, A. M. Abortion, psychiatry, and the quality of life. *American Journal of Psychiatry,* 1972, *128,* 946–951.

Levene, H. I., and Rigney, F. J. Law, preventive psychiatry, and therapeutic abortion. *Journal of Nervous and Mental Disease,* 1970, *151,* 51–59.

Luscutoff, S. A., and Elms, A. C. Advice in the abortion decision. *Journal of Counseling Psychology,* 1975, *22,* 140–146.

Malmquist, A., Kaij, L., and Nilsson, A. Psychiatric aspects of spontaneous abortion: a matched control study of women with living children. *Journal of Psychosomatic Research,* 1969, *13,* 45–59.

Malpas, P. A study of abortion sequences. *Journal of Obstetrics and Gynecology of the British Empire,* 1938, *45,* 932–934.

Mann, E. C. Habitual abortion. *American Journal of Obstetrics and Gynecology,* 1959, *77,* 706.

Margolis, A., Davison, L., Hanson, K., Loos, S. A., and Mikkelsen, C. M. Therapeutic abortion follow-up study. *American Journal of Obstetrics and Gynecology,* 1971, *110,* 243–249.

Meikle, S., Brody, H., Gerritse, R., and Maslany, G. Therapeutic abortion: a prospective study. Part 2. *American Journal of Obstetrics and Gynecology,* 1973, *115,* 339–346.

Meikle, S., Robinson, C., and Brody, H. Recent changes in the emotional reactions of therapeutic abortion applicants. *Canadian Psychiatric Association Journal,* 1977, *22,* 67–70.

Melamed, L. Therapeutic abortion in a midwestern city. *Psychiatric Research Reports,* 1975, *37,* 1143–1146.

Meyerowitz, S., Satloff, A., and Romano, J. Induced abortion for psychiatric indication. *American Journal of Psychiatry,* 1971, *127,* 1153–1160.

Niswander, K. R., and Patterson, R. J. Psychological reactions to abortion: subjective patient responses. *Obstetrics and Gynecology,* 1967, *29,* 702–706.

Niswander, K., Singer, J., and Singer, M. Psychological reactions to therapeutic abortion. Part 2: Objective response. *American Journal of Obstetrics and Gynecology,* 1972, *114,* 29–33.

Ostofsky, H. J., and Ostofsky, J. D. *The abortion experience: Psychological and medical impact.* New York: Harper & Row, 1973.

Pare, C. M., and Raven, H. Follow-up of patients referred for termination of pregnancy. *Lancet,* 1970, *1,* 635–638.

PATT, S. L., RAPPAPORT, R. G., and BARGLOW, P. Follow-up of therapeutic abortion. *Archives of General Psychiatry,* 1969, *20,* 408-414.

PAYNE, E. C., KRAVITZ, A. R., NOTMAN, M. T., and ANDERSON, J. V. Outcome following therapeutic abortion. *Archives of General Psychiatry,* 1976, *33,* 725-733.

PEEK, A., and MARCUS, H. Psychiatric sequelae of therapeutic intervention of pregnancy. *Journal of Nervous and Mental Disease,* 1966, *143,* 417-425.

PEREZ-REYES, M. G., and FALK, R. Follow-up after therapeutic abortion in early adolescence. *Archives of General Psychiatry,* 1973, *28,* 120-126.

ROHT, L. H., and AOYANIA, H. Induced abortion and its sequelae: prematurity and spontaneous abortion. *American Journal of Obstetrics and Gynecology,* 1974, *120,* 868-874.

ROOKS, J. B., and CATES, W., JR. Abortion methods: morbidity, costs, and emotional impact. Part 3: Emotional impact of D and C versus instillation. *Family Planning Perspectives,* 1977, *9,* 276-277.

ROSEN, H. I., SMITH, W. G., and LEBENSOHN, A. M. The quality of life as opposed to the right to life. *American Journal of Psychiatry,* 1972, *129,* 358-360.

ROWINSKY, J. J., and GUSBERG, S. B. Current trends in therapeutic termination of pregnancy. *American Journal of Obstetrics and Gynecology,* 1967, *98,* 11-17.

SCLARE, A. B., and GERAGHTY, B. P. Therapeutic abortion: a follow-up study. *Scottish Medical Journal,* 1971, *16,* 438-442.

———. Therapeutic abortion: a follow-up study. *Psychotherapy and Psychosomatics,* 1972-1973, *21,* 330-331.

SENAY, E. C. Therapeutic abortion. *Archives of General Psychiatry,* 1970, *23,* 408-415.

SIMON, N. M., ROTHMAN, D., GOFF, J. T., and SENTURIA, A. G. Psychological factors related to spontaneous and therapeutic abortion. *American Journal of Obstetrics and Gynecology,* 1969, *104,* 799-806.

SIMON, N. M., SENTURIA, A. G., and ROTHMAN, D. Psychiatric illness following therapeutic abortion. *American Journal of Psychiatry,* 1967, *124,* 97-103.

SMITH, E. M. A follow-up study of women who request abortion. *American Journal of Orthopsychiatry,* 1973, *43,* 574-585.

SQUIER, R., and DUNBAR, F. Emotional factors in the course of pregnancy. *Psychosomatic Medicine,* 1946, *8,* 161-172.

TALAN, K. H., and KIMBAL, C. P. Characterization of 100 women psychiatrically evaluated for therapeutic abortion. *Archives of General Psychiatry,* 1972, *26,* 571-577.

TODD, N. A. Psychiatric experience of the abortion act (1967). *British Journal of Psychiatry,* 1971, *119,* 489-495.

———. Follow-up of patients recommended for therapeutic abortion. *British Journal of Psychiatry,* 1972, *120,* 645-646.

TUPPER, C., MOYA, F., STEWART, L. C., WEIL, R. J., and GRAY, J. D. The problem of spontaneous abortion. Part 1: A combined approach. *American Journal of Obstetrics and Gynecology,* 1957, *73,* 313.

TUPPER, C., and WEIL, R. J. The problem of spontaneous abortion. Part 9: The treatment of habitual aborters by psychotherapy. *American Journal of Obstetrics and Gynecology,* 1962, *83,* 421-424.

VANDENBERGH, R. L., TAYLOR, S., and DROSE, V. Emotional illness in habitual aborters following suturing of the incompetent cervical os. *Psychosomatic Medicine,* 1966, *28,* 257-263.

WALLERSTEIN, J., KURTZ, P., and BAR-DIN, M. Psychosocial sequelae of therapeutic abortion in young unmarried women. *Archives of General Psychiatry,* 1972, *27,* 828-832.

WARBURTON, D., and FRASER, F. C. Genetic aspects of abortion. *Clinical Obstetrics and Gynecology*, 1959, *2*, 22-26.

———. Spontaneous abortion risks in man: data from reproductive histories collected in a medical genetics unit. *American Journal of Human Genetics*, 1964, *16*, 1-5.

WARNES, H. Delayed after effects of medically induced abortion. *Canadian Psychiatric Association Journal*, 1971, *16*, 537-541.

WEIL, R. J., and TUPPER, C. Personality, life situation, and communication: a study of habitual abortion. *Psychosomatic Medicine*, 1960, *22*, 448-455.

WHITTINGTON, H. Evaluation of therapeutic abortion as an element of preventive psychiatry. *American Journal of Psychiatry*, 1970, *126*, 1224-1229.

# PART II

## POSTDELIVERY

# Chapter 4

# The Psychological Factors in Postpartum Reactions

THE BIRTH OF A CHILD produces widespread changes in the family. The parturient woman is suddenly faced with the urgent demands of a new infant while undergoing profound physiological changes. Similarly, fathers, grandparents, and siblings must adjust to the presence of a new family member. Such stresses are presumably not new in our time. Indeed, Hippocrates and Galen described postpartum psychoses ages ago. Although many couples find the birth of a child a rewarding and enriching experience, most of the professional literature has focused on potential problems encountered by the new mother. Consequently, the current discussion will adopt this orientation while keeping in mind that research on the positive aspects of childbirth is badly needed.

In the pre-Freudian mid-nineteenth century postpartum depression and psychoses were well described (Marcé, 1858). The prevailing theory of etiology at that time, not surprisingly, implicated organic causes. More recently attempts have been made (Herzog & Detre, 1976) to meld medical-organic with psychodynamic viewpoints and again to consider postpartum psychiatric illness as a clustering of various psychiatric disorders during the puerperium.

The period around childbirth may be regarded as a time of crisis for the mother (Bibring, 1961). Certainly, the findings that anxiety and tension increase during pregnancy, particularly during the last trimester (discussed in Chapter 1) support this observation. As Karacan and Williams (1970) pointed out, "There has been a widespread feeling among practicing physicians that a certain amount of emotional disturbance is to be expected as a normal consequence of the post-partum period" (p. 308).

Responses to childbirth vary dramatically, in terms of both symptom severity and length of disturbance. As noted, there are women who find childbirth a positive, or only minimally distressing, experience. However, on the other extreme, a small number of women experience frank psychoses during or following childbirth. The overall incidence of adverse or symptomatic responses appears to be inversely related to severity, with psychoses being estimated at 1 in 500 (Herzog & Detre, 1976; Pitt, 1975) a mild, transient mood disturbance, often referred to as the maternity blues, appears to occur in 50% (Pitt, 1973) to 80% (Robbin, 1962) of women following delivery.

The emergence of psychopathology at this time, particularly in the moderate to severe range, is likely to have a detrimental impact on the mother-child relationship. Recent research (described in Chapter 7) has suggested that processes interfering with maternal-infant bonding, especially in the sensitive neonatal period (the first four weeks of life), can measurably affect child development months, and perhaps years, later. The belief that major psychiatric disturbances in new mothers adversely affect child development is widespread but poorly substantiated. Such beliefs are documented by the many child protection laws and agencies in most Western countries. Psychoanalytic theories of the importance of early mothering in the development of childhood and adult psychopathology have promoted widespread concern about the impact of the psychologically disturbed mother on her child. Also, psychoanalytic work has provided one metapsychological framework for understanding postpartum psychiatric illness and its possible effects on children. Indeed, this framework has been the basis for perhaps the most common treatment approach.

Recent phenomenological data have accumulated concerning the effects of maternal psychiatric illness on children. Bahna and Bjerkedal (1974) described significantly decreased birth weights for the children of mothers with neurotic illness during pregnancy. They also documented increased perinatal morbidity and mortality and obstetrical complications in this same group (compared with controls). Paffenbarger (1964) examined the infants of women with prepartum (68) and postpartum (232) psychoses, comparing them with controls (616). Mean gestational age and birth weight were lower in the postpartum psychotic group. Perinatal mortality in this group was twice (six per thousand) that found in the controls (two per thousand).

Harvey (1978) reviewed the literature and found evidence in several sources for increased neurotic symptomotology in mothers of battered infants. He also found evidence of frequent perinatal separation from mother (42% versus 10% for controls) in battered infants. This has bearing on the treatment of postpartum psychiatric illness and suggests that separating the mother from her infant in the perinatal period may have important deleterious effects on the mother-child relationship and perhaps contribute to subsequent battering of infants.

One of the most dreaded effects of maternal illness on children is child murder. Resnick (1969) has characterized two distinct types: neonaticide and filicide. Neonaticide refers to a mother killing her infant within approximately the first 24 hours of life. Filicide refers to murder, by a parent or parents, of an older child. The problem is not rare: according to Resnick (1969), 1 out of every 22 murders committed in the United States in 1966 was that of a child killed by its parent. Harder (1967) reported that in Denmark between 1946 and 1960, one-half of the victims of homicide were children. Resnick (1970) and Brozovsky and Falit (1971) provided evidence that the psychiatric status of mothers who kill their newborns is usually different from that of mothers who murder older children. Mothers committing neonaticide were significantly younger (89% under the age of 25) than those committing filicide (77% over the age of 25). In addition, a large majority of the mothers in the neonaticide group were unmarried whereas nearly 90% of those in the filicide group were married. Most of the mothers in the neonaticide group had concealed the pregnancy even from family members. The neonaticides most commonly occurred immediately following birth and were seen as an attempt to prevent discovery of the pregnancy and infant. Resnick (1970) found that of 37 women committing neonaticide only 17% were psychotic. However, in 131 cases of filicide, approximately two-thirds of the mothers were psychotic. Depression was rare in the neonaticide group but was found in approximately 70% of the filicide group. Concurrent suicide or suicide attempts among the neonaticide group did not occur. However, one-third of the murderers in the filicide group attempted or succeeded in committing suicide in association with the murder.

Button and Reivich (1972) reviewed 42 psychiatric patients for whom obsessions of infanticide were a central psychopathological feature (86% of these were women). In 53% of the women the onset of symptoms occurred in association with parturition (either during the last trimester of pregnancy or within the first six months after delivery). None of these 42 individuals had attempted to kill their children at the time of seeking psychiatric help. Diagnostically, approximately 50% of individuals in the total sample were thought to be schizophrenic. For 26% the diagnosis was a primary affective disorder, depression.

Marked concern about caring for the baby and excessive worry about the infant's health were commonly seen. Of course, such concerns are to some degree normal in new mothers. However, clinical experience suggests that the development of a frank postpartum psychosis resulting in infanticide may be preceded by abnormal concern and worry about the baby's health. This attitude may manifest itself in increasingly frequent emergency visits to the pediatrician or clinic, at which time the mother exhibits unwarranted concern about the child's health. Evaluation of the infant fails to reveal evidence of illness, but the mother continues to feel that "something must be wrong; he's not breathing right; his color isn't good." Recurrent visits occur and each time the mother seems to be less reassured. This may be followed very rapidly by the appearance of frankly delusional beliefs that the child is ill or dying and by the emergence of a psychotic disorder in the mother that may involve the child in a delusional, and frequently paranoid, scheme. Unfortunately, it is easy to miss such early warning signs of the development of this process, particularly if the mother does not return the child to the same physician for these frequent and increasingly desperate visits. There is a tendency, therefore, to miss early detection in mothers who utilize hospital emergency rooms or public clinics rather than private practitioners.

## COMMON CHANGES ASSOCIATED WITH PREGNANCY

In studies of the psychological difficulties associated with childbirth, the hormonal changes accompanying pregnancy and parturition have often been viewed as playing a contributing role. Since such hormonal changes have been widely discussed, it seems advisable to outline the most salient of these shifts at the outset. Perhaps the most obvious changes involve the production of estrogen and progesterone. As Karacan and Williams (1970) pointed out, in the pregnant state the corpus luteum continues to produce estrogen and progesterone, and as the placenta develops, it also produces these hormones. The plasma level of estrogen continues to increase throughout pregnancy until it reaches about 10 times the normal level. Progesterone also increases, with a slow rise during the first trimester and a rapid rise in the second trimester. Levels of progesterone remain quite elevated (compared to those of nonpregnant women) throughout the third trimester. Both estrogen and progesterone levels drop abruptly after parturition, remaining low until menstruation resumes. Herzog and Detre (1976) pointed out that the increases in estrogen and progesterone during pregnancy are associated in time with increases in the production of 17-hydroxycorticosteroids at the tissue level during pregnancy, with an abrupt decline following delivery. However, corticosteroid-binding globulin also nearly doubles. So, the net increase in free cortisol is not huge (Cope, 1972). Further complicating the issue is evidence (Burke & Roulet, 1970) that the normal diurnal variation of serum corticosteroid levels is altered in pregnancy.

As noted by Karacan and Williams (1970), thyroid and anterior pituitary functioning also change as a result of pregnancy and delivery. It is thought that change in pituitary function results in an increased production of several hormones, including thyrotropic hormones. In addition, the placenta itself produces a kind of thyroid-stimulating hormone. Although total plasma thyroxine rises in pregnancy, there is little change in either triiodothyronine (T3) or free thyroxine (T4) levels (Gelder, 1978).

What of the monoamine neurotransmitters currently implicated in the psychopharmacology of schizophrenia and major affective disorders? Decrease in central nervous system activity of norepinephrine, dopamine, serotonin, and other monoamines is the central hypothesis of the so-called monoamine transmitter theory of depression. By contrast, an increase in such activity is suggested in schizophrenia (and perhaps manic) disorders. In some systems progesterone has been shown to have the effect of decreasing monoamine activity or availability by increasing its enzymatic degradation. Although this might have bearing on the occurrence of premenstrual and intragestational depression it would seem to have an effect opposite to that expected to help explain postpartum depression. However, a rebound phenomenon on central nervous system cells sensitized by relatively decreased monoamine neurotransmitter activity in pregnancy (similar to that postulated in the genesis of tardive dyskinesia) could be related to the occurrence of postpartum psychoses.

Coppen, Stein, and Wood (1978) have reviewed their own, and others', work on plasma tryptophan in depression, specifically in postpartum and perimenopausal women. In addition to other monoamine neurotransmitters, 5-hydroxytryptamine (serotonin), has been implicated in the pathophysiology of affective disorders. Tryptophan is a major precursor of central nervous system serotonin. In studies with small numbers of postpartum patients, lowered free plasma tryptophan correlated significantly with increased depressive mood. However, it is too early to draw clinical conclusions from this work.

Finally, a number of other physiological changes implicated in the etiology of postpartum illness occur during pregnancy and the puerperium. Blood loss, blood volume shifts, serum electrolyte changes, lactation and its endocrine changes, sleep stage disturbances, and puerperal infections have all been considered at one time or another. Of all these, generalized infection (sepsis) has emerged over many years of clinical experience as unequivocally etiologic in some puerperal psychoses. This finding is not unexpected, as sepsis from any cause is well known to produce significant mentational changes. These episodes generally resemble delirium or exhibit other definable features of acute organic brain syndromes. The preponderance of clinical experience with the introduction of asepsis, improved obstetrical care and delivery technique, and antibiotic treatment documents the dramatic decrease of sepsis as a major cause of postpartum psychoses.

Although these represent the major biochemical changes discussed in the literature in relation to psychiatric problems associated with childbirth, it should be kept in mind that the mere existence of a change does not establish a causal link with psychiatric symptomatology. Whether these physiological changes represent coincidental but independent events, contributory factors in causation, or prime etiologic factors remains an issue for continued research.

## COMPLAINTS FOLLOWING CHILDBIRTH

In preliminary studies, Melchoir (1975) and Brown (1975) focused on the kinds of problems typically reported by mothers following the birth of a child. Melchoir, in a longitudinal study, observed six women (three primiparas and three multiparas) over the six-week period following childbirth. In the first week postpartum these women identified from 6 to 19 problems, with the most common being physical in nature, e.g., tender episiotomy, abdominal pain, and constipation. Over the next five weeks the range of problems reported decreased so that by the sixth week the number of problems identified varied from 2 to 17. In addition, there appeared to be a shift in the nature of the problems, with physical complaints less prominent and psychological and social problems more so. The latter included feelings of being tied down, concern over the care of the baby, irritability, concern about future pregnancy and methods of family planning, and dyspareunia (painful intercourse).

Looking at a series of informal group discussions with recent mothers, Brown (1975) suggested several factors as being particularly relevant to postpartum adjustment. Lack of sleep during late pregnancy and the first month postpartum was seen as a major contributor to feelings of depression and irritability. Karacan, Heine, Agnew, Williams, Web, and Ross (1968) and Karacan and Williams (1970) have documented the effects of such sleep disturbances in a series of laboratory investigations. In a small sample they found that during late pregnancy there was a substantial reduction in stage four sleep, a reduction in total sleep time, and a significant increase in the number of wakenings. Their results also indicated that sleep patterns did not return to normal until four to six weeks postpartum.

Brown (1975) also reported feelings of anger and resentment experienced by the new mother during the first month postpartum. These feelings appeared to be associated with the requirement for the mother to gear her behavior to the demands of the infant and with her perception of the comparative good health and mobility of the husband. Other issues suggested by Brown included concerns about maternal adequacy and the feeling of not enjoying new motherhood as much as anticipated, based on cultural beliefs and expectations. Trick (1975) has also suggested that discrepancies between actual feelings and cultural expectations may be a significant source of stress for the new mother.

Though the studies by Melchoir (1975) and Brown (1975) had a number of significant methodological shortcomings, e.g., inadequate sample size and lack of suitable control groups, their findings provide some idea of the postpartum problems perceived by recent mothers and demonstrate the potential value of this research approach. Certainly, systematic research into the kinds of difficulties encountered by women following childbirth, the severity of these problems, and the way they are resolved would prove valuable in understanding the psychosocial implications of childbirth.

## SEXUALITY FOLLOWING CHILDBIRTH

One area receiving particular research attention is the sexual activity and responsiveness of women following childbirth. Masters and Johnson (1966), in a longitudinal study of sexual behavior during and after pregnancy, found that half of their respondents reported low levels of sexuality at three months postpartum. Falicov (1973) found that 7 of 19 women had delayed resumption of intercourse beyond two months postpartum. For only half of the remaining 12 couples did sexual adjustment return to prepregnancy levels. Examining interest in intercourse and subjective ratings of the coital orgasmic response, Baxter (1974) found that approximately one-third of the respondents reported increases in both of these measures; approximately another third reported decreases. The final third reported no change from prepregnancy levels during the 11- to fifteen-week period following childbirth. (This is reminiscent of the time-honored clinical dictum that in illnesses for which there is no specific treatment, regardless of what is done, a third get better, a third worse, and a third stay the same.) However, in Falicov's (1973) study, most of the women who had resumed intercourse reported that the achieving of orgasm was more difficult than it had been before pregnancy. The differences between Baxter's and Falicov's results may merely reflect the difference in time since parturition involved in the two studies.

The major reasons for the decreased sexual satisfaction reported by the respondents in the Falicov (1973) study who had not resumed intercourse or who were less satisfied with sex postpartum included fatigue and tension associated with the care of the baby, breast tenderness caused by engorgement, and soreness in the episiotomy site. Some also reported anxiety related to perceived changes in their sexual organs, with vaginal muscles seeming to be either tighter, making intercourse painful, or more slack—a condition they feared might detract from their husband's sexual satisfaction. Interestingly, Baxter (1974) found that the coital orgasm score increased with the perception that the vagina was more slack and decreased with the perception that the vagina was tighter.

Baxter (1974) found no relationship between the coital orgasm score or interest in intercourse and any of the following variables: age, education, social class of the woman's father or husband, age of first boyfriend, age of first intercourse, length of marriage, length of sexual relationship with husband, premarital conception, age at menarche, length of monthly cycle, bleeding time, premenstrual tension syndrome, or dysmenorrhea. There was also no relation to any of the following: vomiting for one week or more, heartburn for two months or more, preeclamptic toxemia including edema only, unplanned pregnancy, sex of the child, or major direction of change in interest in intercourse during pregnancy.

One particularly intriguing finding from the Baxter study was a highly significant positive relationship between increase in the coital orgasm score and the length of the second stage of labor (the period from complete dilatation of the cervix to delivery of the infant). This relationship held up even when controlling for forceps assisted delivery (also positively associated with both increased orgasmic scores and length of second stage of labor). Baxter suggested the common physiological mechanism of uterine contractions in orgasm (Masters & Johnson, 1966) and labor as a possible explanation.

## MATERNITY BLUES

The mildest depressive response postpartum is referred to as the "maternity blues," the "post-baby blues," or the "third-day blues." This syndrome is characterized by a mild to moderate depressive mood lasting from a few hours to several days. Tearfulness and crying, physical discomfort, anxiety about physical health of self and baby, poor concentration, mild confusion, and difficulty in sleeping, along with the mild depressive mood, are the major symptoms (Hamilton, 1962). Yalom, Lunde, Moos, and Hamberg (1968), in a controlled study, found that the maternity blues was specific to childbirth and not merely a function of hospitalization.

The reported incidence of the condition varies widely from one study to another with Oppenheim (1962) reporting an incidence of 15% and Robbin (1962) reporting an incidence of 80%. Most studies, however, report incidence rates between 50% and 70% (Davidson, 1972; Pitt, 1973; Yalom et al., 1968). Variations in reported incidence appear to be primarily the result of differences in definition of the condition and in the time since parturition. Nott, Franklin, Armitage, and Gelder (1976) observed in their sample that emotional upset was common immediately before and immediately after delivery, declining over the ten days following childbirth. Similarly, Pitt (1973) found that the peak incidence of maternity blues occurred on the third day postpartum, with 66% of the women developing it by the fourth day. This lag period, i.e., the peak occurrence of postpartum psychiatric symptoms three or four days after delivery, has been an observed clinical phenomenon for years. It has also served as contributory evidence for the etiologic importance in such symptoms of the impressive drop in plasma estrogens and progesterone postpartum. Levels of these hormones reach their nadir on about day three or four. However, Davidson (1972), in his study of Jamaican women, found a consistent trend for scores on a depressive inventory to decline (i.e., decreased depression) from early in pregnancy into the puerperium. He also noted the similarity between this finding and that of Jarrahi-Zadeh, Kane, Van de Castle, Lachenbruch, and Ewing (1969), who observed that depression was more common in pregnancy than in the postpartum period.

Pitt (1973) and Davidson (1972) examined the reasons for feeling depressed given by mothers experiencing the maternity blues. Among the most frequent reasons given by such mothers in Pitt's study were worries about the baby and difficulties involving breastfeeding. In both studies feelings of homesickness were often cited. Davidson also found that crying because of pain was common. Crying because of pain was less commonly reported in Pitt's sample. Finally, 16% of the women in Pitt's study who experienced the maternity blues could give no reason for their depressed feelings.

Biochemical factors, particularly hormonal, as possibly etiologically important have received some research attention. Stein, Milton, Bebbington, Wood, and Coppen (1976) found a positive correlation between free plasma tryptophan levels and depression in a group of 18 postpartum women. The possible effect of progesterone on plasma tryptophan was described earlier. Nott et al. (1976) examined emotional state as a function of hormonal changes following childbirth. They observed a positive relationship between predelivery estrogen levels and self-rated irritability following parturition. In addition, the greater the drop in progesterone following delivery, the more likely women were to rate themselves as depressed but the less likely to report a sleep disturbance. Finally, the lower the estrogen levels postpartum, the more sleep disturbance was reported. It should be noted that Nott et al. (1976) minimized the overall significance of these findings, pointing out that the significant correlations were of modest proportion (in the range of .30 to .50) and that the other tested relationships did not approach statistical significance.

Looking at personal and social variables, Davidson (1972), in his study of Jamaican women, found that mild postpartum depression was related to ambivalent or hostile feelings toward the baby during the early stages of pregnancy, higher anxiety during the first trimester of pregnancy (as measured by the Maudsley Personality Inventory), and multiparity or subsequent tubal ligations. Pitt (1973) found a greater incidence of difficulty in breastfeeding among new mothers experiencing the maternity blues as compared with new mothers who did not experience this condition. However, Davidson (1972) failed to find any relationship between breastfeeding and the maternity blues. Nott et al. (1976) found that feelings of depression in the immediate puerperium were associated with increased weight gain during the last trimester and with a history of premenstrual tension. Notably, both of these last two variables may involve physiological as well as psychosocial mechanisms. However, Pitt (1973) found no relationship between the maternity blues and menstrual difficulties. In contrast to Davidson (1972), Nott et al. (1976) observed a positive correlation between depressive feelings and primiparity. The discrepancy between these two studies may reflect cultural differences between the Jamaican women studied by Davidson and the British women studied by Nott et al. In addition, Davidson (1972) reported a high incidence of grand multiparity (approximately 33% of the women had five to nine children) in his sample. Finally, it should be noted that Pitt (1973) failed to find any relationship between parity and the occurrence of the maternity blues.

Studies have failed to find a relationship between mild postpartum mood changes and such factors as age (Davidson, 1972; Nott et al., 1976), induced labor, length of labor, experiencing of labor as difficult or painful, extroversion and neuroticism scores at the time of delivery (Nott et al., 1976; Pitt, 1973), health of the neonate (Davidson, 1972; Pitt, 1973), marital status, personal or family history of psychiatric illness, postpartum obstetrical complications, and having a baby of the desired sex (Davidson 1972).

In summary, it appears that the maternity blues represent a rather widespread though not severe syndrome. The condition appears to be specific to childbirth. It would seem that the condition may have some relation to the alteration in hormonal levels experienced around parturition. It may represent a mild, almost subclinical, form of the more severe disorders described in the following sections. The relationship of the condition to personal and social variables is unclear, with contradictory findings frequently reported.

## MODERATELY SEVERE ILLNESS DURING THE PUERPERIUM

A significant number of women appear to experience psychological distress of substantial degree following childbirth. Such syndromes include a variety of neurotic patterns, psychosomatic disorders, brief psychotic episodes, and, most commonly, puerperal depression (Hatrick, 1976; Pitt, 1975; Trick, 1975). Pitt (1968), relying on a prospective study of 300 women, described a condition as marked by depression that lasts over a month and is at least partially disabling. Fatigue, irritability toward the spouse and other children, anxiety especially over the baby, anorexia, insomnia, lack of interest in sex, and feelings of despondency are common features. The degree of depression also appears to vary slightly from day to day and to be generally worse in the evening.

The reported incidence of such a depressive response varies from 6% to 11% of women giving birth (Dalton, 1971; Pitt, 1975). Pitt (1968) found that an additional 6% of his sample experienced psychosomatic symptoms. Nilsson and Almgren (1970), in a prospective study, found that 19% of 165 women had significant psychiatric symptoms within the first six months postpartum. Pitt (1975), reviewing his experience in postnatal clinics, offered the opinion that these estimates reflect only the worst cases and that as many as one-third of postpartum women experience anxiety or depression for a month (or more) of the puerperium. Earlier this same investigator (Pitt, 1968) conducted a follow-up study of puerperal depression. He examined 28 of an initial 33 cases of puerperal depression one year postpartum. Of these, 16 had fully recovered, taking from a few weeks to several months to do so. The remaining 12 women showed no improvement after a year. This unimproved group represented 3.6% of the initial sample of 33 depressed women. This initial sample of puerperal depressive cases differed from the nondepressed control group primarily in terms of premorbid personality, with the depressed individuals appearing more neurotic and less extroverted than the control group. Neither Pitt (1975) nor Dalton (1971) reported a higher incidence of previous psychiatric illness among their cases of moderately severe puerperal depression.

Some investigators have examined postpartum disturbance in relation to psychological changes during pregnancy. Dalton (1971) found among puerperally depressed women a tendency for anxiety and irritability early in pregnancy followed by feelings of elation later in pregnancy. In her study, 64% of puerperally depressed women evidenced elation as compared with 26% of the control women. She found no relationship between such intragestational symptoms as nausea, vomiting, headaches, backaches, or tiredness with subsequent puerperal depression. She suggested that her findings might be related to hormonal variations, citing similar findings from a study on premenstrual tension (Dalton, 1964).

Uddenberg and Nilsson (1975) conducted a somewhat more systematic examination of the relationship of psychological disturbance during pregnancy to postpartum adjustment. They divided their sample into those women who experienced psychological disturbance during pregnancy and those who did not. Overall, they found that those experiencing such distress during pregnancy were more likely to experience adjustment difficulties during the puerperium. In addition, they sought correlates of postpartum adjustment within each of the two groups. Among those showing disturbance during pregnancy, prognosis for the puerperium was worse for those displaying a negative attitude toward future pregnancies, a repudiation of their own mother, and good social circumstances at the time of the pregnancy. For those women not experiencing psychological distress during pregnancy, a poorer prognosis for the puerperium was associated with denial of the pregnancy and denial of somatic sensations connected with it.

When considered as a whole, moderate puerperal depression appears to represent a significant clinical problem in terms of both incidence and degree of disturbance. There is, however, no clear evidence for significantly increased suicide rates in postpartum women. The limited findings available suggest the importance of psychological adjustment during pregnancy as a contributor to this postpartum clinical condition. Clearly, many questions remain concerning these moderately severe disturbances.

## PUERPERAL PSYCHOSIS

The most severe psychiatric disturbance associated with childbirth is referred to as puerperal, or postpartum, psychosis. This is defined as a psychotic episode that occurs during the puerperium. Such conditions tend to be sudden in onset with dramatic psychotic symptomatology. Psychotic episodes are among the earliest recognized psychiatric complications of childbirth, described in antiquity and studied by Esquoril and Marcellus in the nineteenth century. They have received considerable research attention in recent years (Paffenbarger, 1964; Protheroe, 1969; Tod, 1964; Zilboorg, 1957).

The major controversy surrounding puerperal psychosis involves the question of whether it should be regarded as a distinct syndrome or diagnosis separate from other psychiatric illness. Most authors appear to think not. Although specific thought patterns, apparent psychodynamic conflicts, and objects of anxiety, usually centering around the new baby, may be different in puerperal and nonpuerperal psychoses, patients with postpartum psychoses demonstrate the same phenomonologic or descriptive signs and symptoms as patients with acute nonpuerperal psychoses (Herzog & Detre, 1976; Karacan & Williams, 1970).

The reasons presented by the minority of authors and clinicians who continue to consider these illnesses as distinct psychopathological entities are given here.

1. Timing—onset rarely before the third day postpartum (i.e., the lag, or latent, period), suggesting a relationship to the precipitous estrogen and progesterone reductions of this period.
2. Onset of symptoms—ususually preceded by a specific pattern of clinical signs including depressed and/or labile affect and irritability.
3. Reports of associated reproductive pathology—menstrual irregularities, premenstrual symptoms, with occasionally successful progesterone therapy.
4. Reports of thyroid dysfunction—changes in free thyroxine and successful treatment of some postpartum psychotic syndromes with thyroid replacement (Karacan & Williams, 1970).
5. Evidence of organic brain dysfunction—confusion, disorientation,

delirium in a significant number of cases; change in the incidence of such manifestations with modern improvements in obstetrical care.

6. Psychodynamic formulations—years of case reports and psychoanalytically oriented studies describing specific psychological conflicts associated with pregnancy, childbirth, separation and individuation, and mothering in women with such psychoses (these include reports of successful treatment using therapeutic techniques derived from psychoanalytic theory).

However, Swift (1972) has argued that the factors most frequently cited in the etiology of puerperal psychoses are the same factors normally cited to explain most psychiatric illness, i.e., latent psychosis or predisposition to psychosis, psychologically stressful precipitants, as well as toxic and metabolic factors. In short, the primary reasons for continuing to use the terms "postpartum psychosis" or "puerperal psychosis" are probably historical and practical (the psychosis happens to occur in the puerperium).

## Forms of Puerperal Psychosis

Postpartum psychoses are usefully phenomenologically classified as affective, schizophrenic, or organic disorders. The last diagnosis has become less frequent as obstetrical practices have improved (Tetlow, 1955). At present (Ebie, 1972; Gupta & Agarwal, 1975), organic postpartum psychoses are most often reported in geographical areas where modern obstetrical medicine is not available.

In a study of 224 women who had psychotic illnesses associated with childbirth, from a total of 1295 woman admitted to a mental hospital, Stevens (1971) found severe depression and schizophrenia to be the most prevalent forms of psychosis, with depression comprising the greater percentage. However, some studies done in the United States have shown a preponderance of schizophrenia among postpartum psychotics. This may be related to the often mentioned observation that affective disorders are underdiagnosed in the United States (as compared with Britain) or to the decreased severity of illness in affective disease, resulting in fewer hospitalizations (Herzog & Detre, 1976). Studies conducted in England have shown that affective illness is diagnosed more often than schizophrenia in postpartum women in that country.

## Incidence

The incidence of psychosis associated with childbirth as reported in the literature has generally ranged from 1 in 400 births (Herzog & Detre, 1976) to 1 in 500 births (Pitt, 1975). In their review of the literature, Herzog and Detre (1976) reported that 2-8% of female admissions to mental hospitals are diagnosed as having a postpartum psychosis. The differences in reported incidence most probably reflect differences in diagnostic criteria.

The reported incidence of postpartum psychoses has decreased since the 1950s. This trend is generally attributed to the introduction of antibiotics in the treatment of puerperal infection. Before 1945, most studies quoted 20–50% of postpartum psychiatric conditions as having a toxic cause. Since that time, toxic and septic episodes postpartum resulting from infection, and the accompanying organic psychotic syndromes, have dramatically decreased (Tetlow, 1955). However, clinical experience documents that transient organic confusional states, without fully developed delirium or psychosis, continue to occur not infrequently even with modern obstetrical care. These episodes are generally not labeled or diagnosed as postpartum psychiatric disturbances for two reasons: (1) they are usually quite brief and (2) the underlying obstetrical problem causing the mentational disturbance (e.g., sepsis or hypoxia) is the diagnostic label applied.

## Onset

The greatest percentage (45%) of puerperal psychotic episodes occur in the first two weeks postpartum (Herzog & Detre, 1976), but psychotic episodes of any degree of severity can occur up to six months postpartum. Prodromal manifestations develop around the third day. Pitt (1975) found that the onset of mild disturbance occurred about the third or fourth day postpartum; moderate depressive and anxiety states between delivery and six weeks; and psychosis anywhere between delivery and six months.

## Prognosis

In general, patients with puerperal psychoses have the same long-term prognosis as patients with nonpuerperal psychoses of the same phenomenologic type, i.e., affective, schizophrenic, or organic (Baker et al., 1971; Herzog & Detre, 1976; Wilson, Barglow, & Shipman, 1972). In general, long-term prognosis is poorer for (1) patients manifesting schizophrenic, rather than affective, symptomatology and (2) patients with a history of psychiatric illness, postpartum or not. However, patients with bipolar manic-depressive illness are twice as likely as other psychotics to have postpartum recurrences; moreover, such a recurrent psychotic episode is three and a half times more likely during the puerperium than during any other time in the patient's life after 15 years of age. Indeed, the high frequency of recurrence of bipolar illness during the puerperium has been used to support the theory that postpartum psychosis is a distinct entity.

In a long-term follow-up study of 134 patients with postpartum psychosis, Protheroe (1969) found that 35 years later, 78% of affective, and 30% of schizophrenic, patients were at home and symptom-free. Another 30% of schizophrenic patients never left the hospital after the original illness, whereas the remainder were at home but had residual symptoms. (This is another example of the so-called rule of thirds mentioned earlier in this chapter.) Thirteen percent of all patients had experienced another postpartum psychosis; 39% had a nonpuerperal psychotic episode at some later time; and 5% had both. Although the schizophrenic prognosis was more grave, this study found no greater susceptibility to recurrent postpartum episodes in the schizophrenic than in the affective group (Protheroe, 1969).

## Individual Characteristics

Age. The average age of women at the onset of psychosis associated with childbirth is 28 years, with most illness occurring in women between 22 and 28 years of age and rarely occurring in women under 20 or over 40 (Herzog & Detre, 1976). It must be kept in mind, however, that more babies are born to this age group than to any other and a comparison of postpartum women with women not recently delivered, but of comparable age, revealed a similar incidence of psychosis (Paul, 1974).

Marital Status. Ten to fifteen percent of women with puerperal psychosis are single (Herzog & Detre, 1976). According to most authors extramarital conception does not appear to contribute to puerperal illness (Paul, 1974). However, Kendell (1978) found that 22% of 99 women developing psychiatric illness had given birth to illegitimate children in the studied period (this is twice the rate expected). This review included nonpuerperal as well as postpartum illness. Kendell concluded that there is an association between illegitimate pregnancy and psychiatric illness but that the illness is as likely to precede as to follow the pregnancy. Among patients having illegitimate babies the preponderant psychotic type appears to be schizophrenic. Stevens (1971) studied 224 women admitted to a London hospital with puerperal psychosis. She found in this sample that puerperal depression was more frequent than puerperal schizophrenia, perhaps because of the higher fertility rate of the depressives. The unmarried women in her sample had a greater incidence (twice) of schizophrenia than of depression. (It is of note that women with nonpuerperal schizophrenic syndromes have significantly lower marriage and reproductive rates than do women with affective illness.)

Parity. Most studies have found that primiparas are more likely than multiparas to experience a psychosis associated with childbirth (Herzog & Detre, 1976; Paul, 1974). Fifty to 66% of all puerperal psychoses occur in primiparous women. One study (Paul, 1974) documented that 50% of postpartum psychotics were primiparous during a period when primiparas accounted for only one-third of the deliveries. However, the first episode of psychosis associated with childbirth can occur with any pregnancy.

History and Heredity. A history of psychiatric illness is reported for about 30% of both puerperal and nonpuerperal psychotic women (Dalton, 1971; Herzog & Detre, 1976; Pitt, 1968).

Researchers have attempted to determine the role of heredity in postpartum psychosis. Thuwe (1974), in noting the occurrence of mental illness among all children and grandchildren of a group of women undergoing a first episode of postpartum psychosis within six weeks of childbirth, found that a history of mental illness or psychiatric treatment in the children of these women was significantly more common than chance would have dictated. This propensity was not statistically significant in the grandchildren. Although these findings may be consistent with an environmental explanation (i.e., the influence of a mother who has had a psychotic episode), the cases of psychosis in the child generation were distributed in such a way as to make the environmental hypothesis improbable. That is, the affected children (a total of 28) were born to only 20 of the total of 43 women whose children had reached adult age.

In this same study, subjects were identified by social group. Surprisingly, the affected children and their mothers clustered in the higher social levels. An environmental hypothesis is hard-pressed to explain this increased incidence of psychiatric disturbance or treatment in individuals of higher socioeconomic status (compared with those in lower social levels). The presumably improved socioeconomic conditions would be thought to decrease morbidity. However, diagnosis of psychiatric illness, and its treatment, may be artificially increased in the upper socioeconomic group because of availability of mental health services and because of attitudinal differences affecting the use of such services.

First-degree relatives of postpartum psychotics have been found to have a 14% lifetime incidence of mental illness (Herzog & Detre, 1976). Although this figure is higher than that for the general population, it is about the same as that for nonpuerperal psychotics. It can be argued, therefore, that heredity plays some part in the predisposition to puerperal mental illness but probably no greater a role than in nonpuerperal psychosis.

Biology. A lag period of two days immediately following childbirth (when the occurrence of a psychotic episode is relatively rare), coupled with the known hormonal changes taking place at this time, suggests to some investigators that endocrine factors contribute to puerperal psychosis. As described, the most common among such etiological theories are those that focus on estrogen and progesterone. The drastic reduction of these hormones postpartum is thought to affect mentation (Dalton, 1971; Herzog & Detre, 1976). A decrease in the production of corticosteroids postpartum has also been cited as an endocrine related cause of postpartum psychotic illness. Studies conducted during pregnancy have noted elation of mood during periods when levels of progesterone, estrogen, and corticosteroids are highest (Dalton, 1971; Herzog & Detre, 1976). Some endocrinological theories having less acceptance have been advanced. Treadway, Kane, Duke, and Lipton (1968) have suggested that catecholamines may play a contributing role. Butts (1968) hypothesized that hypothyroidism plays a part in puerperal psychological disturbance in some cases.

An interesting phenomenon has been reported with regard to the sex of the offspring of women experiencing psychotic episodes postpartum: fewer males (fewer than expected by chance alone) are born to patients who develop a schizophrenic psychosis within one month after childbirth. Schearer, Davidson, and Finch (1967) concluded that in schizophrenic women a serum factor is present that is toxic to the sex chromosome, either in the sperm or fertilized ovum or during the first month of gestation. However, Schorer (1972) examined 36 female schizophrenics whose disorders were temporarily related to pregnancy. No relationship was found between the sex of the offspring and the period (first, second, or third trimester and the puerperium) during which the schizophrenia developed. In addition, the neonatal deaths showed no unusual pattern.

In summary, no clinically useful biological predictors of risk for postpartum psychoses have been found. It is of particular note that no endocrinological markers for such predictions have been identified in spite of current conventional wisdom that endocrine factors are etiologically important.

## Psychogenic Factors

Most authors agree that the period following childbirth is one of stress even for the well-adjusted woman. Conflicts over acceptance of the feminine role, of which mothering is a part, and over the responsibility mothering involves are present for nearly every woman who has a child. Such conflict is sometimes seen as causing a reactivation of earlier developmental difficulties (especially those centering on mother). Hostility toward the baby is thought to be a result of demands, both fantasied and real, on the new mother, demands that she is unwilling or unable to meet. The birth of a baby also may activate conflict with the husband and with other children.

Much of the earlier research into the psychological factors in puerperal psychosis proceeded from a psychodynamic orientation. Brew and Seidenberg (1950), for instance, described psychotically depressed puerperal women who had a narcissistic psychological organization, who were overdependent on their own parents for protection, and who were oversolicitous toward the newborn. Zilboorg (1957) studied postpartum schizophrenics and viewed them as schizoid, sexually frigid, emotionally rigid, and latently homosexual. Martin (1958), however, in a study of 15 postpartum schizophrenics, could not document a schizoid, premorbid personality in 14 of his patients.

In an attempt to determine the role of prior personality in postpartum psychosis, Rosenwald and Stonehill (1972) classified 26 puerperally psychotic women into early and late (after childbirth) admissions to psychiatric in-patient units. They found that those admitted early showed greater lifelong social withdrawal and thought disturbance; later admissions appeared to be more dependent, egocentric, manipulative, and depressed. These differences were statistically reliable and were based on systematic ratings of life history information. They suggested that the early group centered conflicts around the process of having babies, whereas the late group experienced conflicts around the role of mothering.

It seems clear that psychogenic factors are more important than other variables in the etiology of mental illness reported in persons other than the natural mother who become psychotic as a reaction to childbirth. Specifically, there is documentation of psychoses in new grandmothers (Roth, 1975), new fathers, and new adoptive mothers (Asch & Rubin, 1974). If this process can occur in relatives of the mother, how much more important are psychogenic factors in the mothers themselves?

## SUMMARY

Certainly there is no one cause for all postpartum psychoses. Rather, several etiologic factors work together. The puerperium is a period of stress, both physical and psychological, for all mothers. Marked physiological changes occur during this time. If we add to these biological predisposition, a poor relationship with family (especially mother), a previous experience of mental illness, increased incidence of mental illness in first-degree relatives, and personality problems prior to childbirth, the chances for severe postpartum psychological problems are greatly increased.

### Treatment

Mild to moderate postpartum psychiatric syndromes generally require and receive no treatment. Thus, most knowledge of treatment centers on postpartum psychoses. In general, the best treatment for a puerperal psychosis is that which would be undertaken for the same type (phenomenologically) of nonpuerperal psychotic episode. Such treatment usually includes a combination of psychotropic medications (antipsychotic and/or antidepressant), psychotherapy (often with an emphasis on a psychoanalytic or a family approach), and occasionally electroconvulsive therapy. Since these therapeutic modalities have received extensive clinical and research attention in the treatment of all forms of psychoses and since there is no evidence that they are differentially effective for puerperal psychoses, no attempt will be made to review them within the present context. Discussion here will focus on treatment approaches specially designed for puerperal psychoses and on research that has examined the specific response of such patients to these treatments. With this focus it soon becomes apparent that the literature is scanty.

In studies of the response of puerperally psychotic women to hospitalization, Nilsson, Uddenberg, and Almgren (1971) and Wilson and associates (1972) found that an onset of symptoms more than three weeks postpartum and a discharge diagnosis of neurotic depression correlated with good short-term prognosis and good outcome of hospitalization. Brief hospitalization was found to be related to *no* history of treated psychiatric illness prior to pregnancy, the presence of physical problems during pregnancy, delivery, or postpartum, reintegration within the first 10 days of hospitalization, and a discharge diagnosis of neurotic depression. Hormonal therapies have been employed in the treatment of some postpartum psychiatric conditions. Wakoh and Hatotani (1973) found that endocrinological therapy using thyroid hormones, anterior pituitary hormones, ovarian hormones, and adrenocorticoids exerted a marked effect on postpartum psychotics who failed to respond to other types of treatment and who exhibited features of thyroid and adrenocorticoid hypofunction. Furthermore, they found that the effectiveness of electroconvulsive therapy for puerperal depression increased after hormonal therapy. Dalton (1971) reported good results with hormonal therapy for less severe forms of depression following childbirth. Pitt (1975), however, noted that although such studies have reported favorable results with the use of hormonal therapies, these methods have not gained widespread acceptance in the treatment of postpartum conditions. Coppen, Stein, and Wood (1978), although describing a relationship between decreased plasma tryptophan levels postpartum and increased depression, did not cite evidence of successful clinical use of tryptophan in treating postpartum illness. However, Walinder, Skott, and Nagy (1973) did find tryptophan therapy useful in nonpuerperally depressed patients also receiving conventional antidepressant medications.

Psychotherapeutic treatment has traditionally involved a focus on presumed psychodynamic conflicts associated with motherhood, separation, individuation, and childrearing. Early on, individual psychoanalytically oriented psychotherapy was usually employed. However, family therapy, or at least a family systems approach in an individual therapy situation, is increasingly common in recent years.

One treatment strategy involves the joint admission of mother and baby to a psychiatric therapeutic milieu. As described by Brian (1975), in its most ideal form, a homelike atmosphere is created with a small (fewer than 10) number of patients and their babies. A therapeutic community is established in which chores are shared among patients and staff and in which nurses can teach the new mothers how to care for their babies. This relaxed and supportive environment allows the mother to interact freely with her child with professional staff providing assistance or relief whenever necessary.

Mester, Klein, and Lowental (1975) pointed out that this treatment is intended to complement other forms of therapy. These authors suggested that the primary benefit of the therapeutic environment is that it allows the mother and baby to be together during the first stages of the baby's (extrauterine) life so that feelings of maternal love, attachment, and competence can occur under the relatively secure conditions of the hospital.

An insufficient number of studies has been conducted on the effectiveness of this treatment program, but verbal reports by hospital staff and mothers have indicated satisfaction with the program (Luepker, 1972; Mester, Klein, & Lowental, 1975). A study conducted by Lindsay (1975), using readmission as a criterion, found that this mother-baby in-patient treatment program was at least as effective as any other.

## Prevention

Given the extent of various postpartum psychological difficulties, as well as their predictability in time, it would seem that this clinical problem would be a prime target for preventive measures. Relatively little effort, however, has been focused on this area.

Preparing women for childbirth would seem to be the first step in such a preventive program. The prevailing belief in the value of education in preventive medicine suggests that women poorly prepared for labor, delivery, and motherhood experience bewilderment and fear, which contribute to poor adjustment postpartum. Since primiparas seem to be at greater risk (perhaps conflict over the mothering role is most severe for first babies), education to prepare new mothers for delivery and infant care seems a worthwhile approach. An educational program for family members, emphasizing the emotional and practical problems for the new mother, as well as training in the care of the infant, might prove effective in promoting a smooth transition from hospital to home for the parturient woman. The procedure of rooming-in, which allows mother and baby to be together in a maternity ward, might also contribute to prevention.

Pitt (1975), reviewing treatment approaches to postpartum psychological disturbances, described the work of Gordon and Gordon (1960) and Gordon, Kapostins, and Gordon (1965). They found that systematic education of expectant mothers reduced psychiatric morbidity postpartum. The best results appeared to be obtained when (1) husbands attended with their wives; (2) personal and social resources were mobilized during the early puerperium; and (3) women arranged daily tasks to maintain their outside interests. However, health education and the employment of psychoanalytic theory in designing public school curricula (and in other public institutions for the care of children and adults) have not reduced the incidence of schizophrenia or manic-depressive psychoses in the general population over the past 40 years. It seems naive to expect that similar programs will rapidly reduce the incidence of postpartum psychoses. Indeed, psychoanalytic theory suggests that if psychodynamic conflict contributes significantly to postpartum psychiatric illness, health education programs for adolescent or adult women will not reduce postpartum psychiatric morbidity in the overall population. Intensive intervention would have to be made in early childhood or in earlier generations.

Without clear evidence for specific factors, biological or psychological, that contribute in comprehensible ways to the etiology of postpartum psychosis, preventive techniques will remain ineffective.

## CONCLUSION

In reviewing the literature on postpartum psychiatric conditions, several authors (Brown & Shereshefsky, 1972; Karacan et al., 1970) have noted a number of methodological shortcomings common to these studies. These authors reported that many of the published papers were retrospective studies based on records of patients admitted to psychiatric hospitals, thus relying on data that were themselves interpretations. Furthermore, the use of control groups has been infrequent, and even when such have been used they have often not been drawn from the same social and economic levels as the postpartum cases. Though these methodological criticisms continue to be relevant, the soundness of research in the area seems to be improving.

Future research efforts need to employ multifactorial designs in which the influence of several relevant variables can be assessed. Such studies need to adopt prospective, longitudinal strategies and to follow a large sample of women from conception through the puerperium, with later life follow-up. Studies need to be designed in which the overall psychological functioning of the woman is taken into account. Finally, the role of interpersonal factors previously little studied, such as the relationship between the prospective mother and father, needs to be assessed. Of course, studies seeking biological clues must continue. Although existing research has provided important insights into puerperal psychiatric syndromes, it appears that a thorough understanding awaits considerable additional research. Only with such an understanding can sound treatment and prevention programs be designed and implemented.

## REFERENCES

Arboleda-Flores, J. Neonaticide. *Canadian Psychiatric Association Journal,* 1976, *21,* 31–34.

Asch, S., and Rubin, L. Postpartum reactions: some unrecognized variations. *American Journal of Psychiatry,* 1974, *131,* 870–874.

Astrup, C. Maternal schizophrenia and the sex of offspring. *Biological Psychiatry,* 1974, *9,* 211–214.

Bahna, S. L., and Bjerkedal, T. The course and outcome of pregnancy in women with neuroses. *Acta Obstetricia et Gynecologica et Scandinavica,* 1974, *53,* 129–133.

Baker, M., Dorzab, J., Winokur, G., and Cadoret, R. Depressive disease: the effect of the postpartum state. *Biological Psychiatry,* 1971, *3,* 357–365.

BAXTER, S. Labor and orgasm in primipara. *Journal of Psychosomatic Research,* 1974, *18,* 209-216.

BIBRING, G. A study of the psychological processes in pregnancy and of the earliest mother-child relationship. *Psychoanalytic Study of the Child,* 1961, *16,* 9-45.

BREW, M., and SEIDENBERG, R. Psychotic reactions associated with pregnancy and childbirth. *Journal of Nervous and Mental Diseases,* 1950, *111,* 408-423.

BRIAN, V. Postnatal depression. *Nursing Mirror,* 1975, *140,* 68.

BROWN, C. Baby blues. *Nursing Mirror,* 1975, *141,* 61-62.

BROWN, W., and SHERESHEFSKY, P. Seven women: a prospective study of postpartum psychiatric disorders. *Psychiatry,* 1972, *35,* 139-59.

BROZOVSKY, M., and FALIT, H. Neonaticide: clinical and psychodynamic perspectives. *Journal of the American Academy of Child Psychiatry,* 1971, *10,* 673-683.

BURKE, C. W., and ROULET, F. Increased exposure of tissues to cortisol in late pregnancy. *British Medical Journal,* 1970, *1,* 657-659.

BUTTON, J. H., and REIVICH, R. S. Obsessions of infanticide. *Archives of General Psychiatry,* 1972, *27,* 235-240.

BUTTS, H. Psychodynamic and endocrine factors in postpartum psychoses. *Journal of the National Medical Association,* 1968, *60,* 224-227.

COPE, C. L. The adrenal in pregnancy. In *Adrenal steroids and disease* (2d ed.). G. Smith (ed.), London: Pitman, 1972.

COPPEN, A., STEIN, A., and WOOD, K. Postnatal depression and tryptophan metabolism. In M. Sandler (ed.), *Mental illness in pregnancy and the puerperium.* New York: Oxford University Press, 1978.

DALTON, K. The influence of menstruation on health and disease. *Practitioner,* 1964, *192,* 287-288.

———. Puerperal and premenstrual depression. *Proceedings of the Royal Society of Medicine,* 1971, *64,* 1249-1252.

DAVIDSON, J. Postpartum mood change in Jamaican women: a description and discussion of its significance. *British Journal of Psychiatry,* 1972, *121,* 659-663.

EBIE, J. Psychiatric illness in the puerperium among Nigerians. *Tropical Geographic Medicine,* 1972, *24,* 253-256.

FALICOV, C. Sexual adjustment during first pregnancy and post partum. *American Journal of Obstetrics and Gynecology,* 1973, *117,* 991-1000.

GELDER, M. Hormones and post-partum depression. In M. Sandler (ed.), *Mentu. illness in pregnancy and the puerperium.* New York: Oxford University Press, 1978.

GORDON, R., and GORDON, K. Social factors in prevention of postpartum emotional problems. *Obstetrics and Gynecology,* 1960, *15,* 433-438.

GORDON, R., KAPOSTINS, E., and GORDON, K. Factors in postpartum emotional adjustment. *Obstetrics and Gynecology,* 1965, *25,* 158-166.

GUPTA, O., and AGARWAL, S. Psychiatric illness in the puerperium. *Journal of the Indian Medical Association,* 1975, *65,* 45-46.

HAMILTON, J. *Postpartum psychiatric problems.* St. Louis: Mosby, 1962.

HARDER, T. The psychopathology of infanticide. *Acta. Psychiatrica Scandanavica,* 1967, *43,* 196-245.

HARVEY, D. Maternal mental illness: the effects on the baby. In M. Sandler (ed.), *Mental illness in pregnancy and the puerperium.* New York: Oxford University Press, 1978.

HATRICK, J. Puerperal mental illness. *Nursing Times,* 1976, *72,* 533-534.

HERZOG, A., and DETRE, T. Psychotic reactions associated with childbirth. *Diseases of the Nervous System,* 1976, *37,* 229-235.

Jarrahi-Zadeh, A., Kane, F., Van de Castle, R., Lachenbruch, P., and Ewing, J. Emotional and cognitive changes in pregnancy and early puerperium. *British Journal of Psychiatry,* 1969, *115,* 797–805.

Karacan, I., Heine, W., Agnew, H., Williams, R., Web, W., and Ross, J. Characteristics of sleep patterns during late pregnancy and the postpartum period. *American Journal of Obstetrics and Gynecology,* 1968, *101,* 570–586.

Karacan, I., and Williams, R. Current advances in theory and practice relating to postpartum syndromes. *Psychiatry in Medicine,* 1970, *1,* 307–328.

Karnosh, L., and Hope, J. Puerperal psychoses and their sequelae. American Journal of Psychiatry, 1937, *94,* 537–550.

Kendell, R. E. Childbirth as an aetiological agent. In M. Sandler (ed.), *Mental illness in pregnancy and the puerperium.* New York: Oxford University Press, 1978.

Kendell, R. E., Wainwright, S., Hailey, A., and Shannon, B. The influence of childbirth on psychiatric morbidity. Psychological medicine, 1976, *6,* 297–302.

Lewis, P., Ironside, W., McKinnon, P., and Simons, C. The Karitane project: psychological ill-health, infant distress, and the postpartum period. *New Zealand Medical Journal,* 1974, *79,* 1005–1009.

Lindsay, J. Puerperal psychosis: a follow-up study of a joint mother and baby treatment programme. *Australian and New Zealand Journal of Psychiatry,* 1975, *9,* 73–76.

Luepker, E. Joint admission and evaluation of postpartum psychiatric patients and their infants. *Hospital and Community Psychiatry,* 1972, *23,* 284–286.

Marcé, L. U. Traité de la foue des femmes enceintes, des nourvelles accouchées, et des nourrices (Paris, 1858). Cited in F. J. Kane, Jr. Post-partum disorders. In A. M. Freedman, H. I. Kaplan, and B. J. Sadock (eds.), *Comprehensive texbook of psychiatry,* Vol. 2 (2nd ed.). Baltimore: Williams & Wilkins, 1975.

Martin, M. Puerperal mental illness: a follow-up study of 75 cases. *British Medical Journal,* 1958, *2,* 773.

Masters, W., and Johnson, V. *Human sexual response.* Boston: Little, Brown, 1966.

Melchior, L. Is the postpartum period a time of crisis for some mothers? *Canadian Nurse,* 1975, *71,* 30–32.

Melges, F. T. Post-partum psychiatric syndromes. *Psychosomatic Medicine,* 1968, *30,* 95–108.

Mester, R., Klein, H., and Lowental, U. Conjoint hospitalization of mother and baby. *Israel Annals of Psychiatry and Related Disciplines,* 1975, *13,* 124–136.

Nilsson, A., Uddenberg, N., and Almgren, P. E., Parental relations and identification in women with special regard to para-natal emotional adjustment. *Acta Psychiatrica Scandinavica,* 1971, *47,* 57–81.

Nilsson, A., and Almgren, P. Para-natal emotional adjustment: a prospective investigation of 165 women. Part 2: The influence of background factors, psychiatric history, parental relations, and personality characteristics. *Acta Psychiatrica Scandinavica,* 1970, *220,* 65–141.

Nott, P., Franklin, M., Armitage, C., and Gelder, M. Hormonal changes and mood in the puerperium. *British Journal of Psychiatry,* 1976, *128,* 379–383.

Oppenheim, G. Psychological aspects of pregnancy and childbirth. Lecture presented to the Royal Medicopsychological Association, City, 1962.

Paffenbarger, R. Epidemiological aspects of parapartum mental illness. *British Journal of Preventive Social Medicine,* 1964, *18,* 189–195.

Paul, O. A study of puerperal psychosis. *Journal of the Indian Medical Association,* 1974, *63,* 84–89.

PITT, B. Atypical depression following childbirth. *British Journal of Psychiatry,* 1968, *114,* 1325–1335.

———. Maternity blues. *British Journal of Psychiatry,* 1973, *122,* 531–533.

———. Psychological reactions to childbirth. *Proceedings of the Royal Society of Medicine,* 1975, 223–224.

———. Psychiatric illness following childbirth. *British Journal of Psychiatry,* 1975, (special number 9), 409–415.

PROTHEROE, C. A long term study, 1927–1961. *British Journal of Psychiatry,* 1969, *115,* 9–30.

RESNICK, P. J. Child murder by parents: a psychiatric review of filicide. American Journal of Psychiatry 1969, *126,* 325–333.

———. Murder of the newborn: a psychiatric review of neonaticide. American Journal of Psychiatry 1970, *126,* 1414–1420.

ROBBIN, A. Psychological changes of normal parturition. *Psychiatric Quarterly,* 1962, *36,* 129–150.

ROSENWALD, G., and STONEHILL, M. Early and late postpartum illness. *Psychosomatic Medicine,* 1972, *34,* 129–137.

ROTH, N. The mental content of puerperal psychoses. *American Journal of Psychotherapy,* 1975, *29,* 204–211.

SCHEARER, M., DAVIDSON, R., and FINCH, S. The sex ratio of offspring born to state hospitalized schizophrenic women. *Journal of Psychiatric Research,* 1967, *5,* 349–350.

SCHORER, C. Gestational schizophrenia. *Canadian Psychiatric Association Journal,* 1972, *17* (supplement 2), SS 259.

STEIN, G., MILTON, F., BEBBINGTON, P., WOOD, K., and COPPEN, A. Relationship between mood disturbances and free and total plasma tryptophan in postpartum women. *British Medical Journal,* 1976, *2,* 457.

STEVENS, B. Psychoses associated with childbirth: a demographic survey since the development of community care. *Social Science and Medicine,* 1971, *5,* 527–543.

SWIFT, C. Psychosis during the puerperium among Tanzanians. *East African Medical Journal,* 1972, *49,* 651–657.

TAYLOR, M. Sex ratios of newborns and schizophrenia. *Science,* 1970, *168,* 151–152.

TETLOW, C. Psychoses of childbearing. *Journal of Mental Science,* 1955, *101,* 629.

THUWE, I. Genetic factors in puerperal psychosis. *British Journal of Psychiatry,* 1974, *125,* 378–385.

TOD, E. Puerperal depression. *Lancet,* 1964, *2,* 1264.

TREADWAY, R., KANE, F., DUKE, R., and LIPTON, M. A psycho-endocrine study of pregnancy and the puerperium. Paper presented to the American Psychological Association, Boston, 1968.

TRICK, K. Psychological problems following birth and miscarriage. *Nursing Mirror,* 1975, *141,* 61–62.

UDDENBERG, N., and NILSSON, L. The longitudinal course of para-natal emotional disturbance. *Acta Psychiatrica Scandinavica,* 1975, *52,* 160–169.

WAKOH, T., and HATOTANI, N. Endocrinological treatment of psychoses. In K. Lissak (ed.), *Hormones and brain function.* New York: Plenum, 1973.

WALINDER, J., SKOTT, A., NAGY, A., CARLSON, A., ROOS, B. Potentiation of antidepressant action of clomipramine by tryptophan. *Lancet,* 1973, *0,* 984.

WILSON, J., BARGLOW, P., and SHIPMAN, W. The prognosis of postpartum mental illness. *Comprehensive Psychiatry,* 1972, *13,* 305–316.

YALOM, I., LUNDE, D., MOOS, R., and HAMBERG, D. "Postpartum blues" syndrome: a description and related variables. *Archives of General Psychiatry,* 1968, *18,* 16–27.

ZILBOORG, G. The clinical issues of postpartum psychopathological reaction. *American Journal of Obstetrics and Gynecology,* 1957, *73,* 305–312.

ZINNEMAN, H., SEALS, U., and DOE, R. Urinary amino acids in pregnancy, following progesterone, and estrogen-progesterone. *Journal of Clinical Endocrinology and Metabolism,* 1967, *27,* 397–405.

# Chapter 5

# Psychological Reactions to Preterm Birth

THIS CHAPTER FOCUSES ON the situation in which parents are faced with the unexpectedly early birth of an expected child. Whether a child is wanted or not, expectant parents are aware that a birth will occur, and attending physicians usually provide the expectant mother with a due date, a specified time period during which the probability of birth is highest.

In this chapter we will review the rather varied terminology used to characterize preterm births and we will examine the general characteristics of preterm births, but our primary goal is to discuss the literature on parental postpartum reaction to the premature birth of a child. We end the chapter with some general conclusions and recommendations.

## PRETERM BIRTH: TERMINOLOGY AND GENERAL CHARACTERISTICS

It is clearly beyond the scope of this text exhaustively to examine the utility and medical import of the various diagnostic categories and terms that have been proposed as useful in the classification of preterm births and other varieties of gestational irregularity. Because of the range of terms proposed, and the different operational definitions of the same term, it is necessary to discuss the problem briefly.

In the popular press, *premature* is probably the word most often used to describe infants born "too soon." In medical and psychological practice, however, a wide variety of terms, designed to designate identical or closely related conditions, have appeared in the professional literature of recent years: low birth weight, prematurity, immaturity, preterm, term, postterm, dysmaturity, small for date, and so on (American Academy of Pediatrics, 1967; Gruenwald, 1974; Hellman & Pritchard, 1971; Korones, Lancaster, & Roberts, 1972; Lesser, 1973; Paton & Fisher, 1973; Ritz, 1975; Scipien et al., 1975). The greatest degree of ambiguity has been in the use of the terms *low birth weight, preterm,* and *premature.* All three of these apply to infants who at birth are small or puny, who exhibit a variety of symptoms that distinguish them from other babies, and who tend to weigh significantly less than so-called normal infants. Although the diagnostic labels clearly delineate different syndromes, the ambiguity has arisen because practitioners and researchers have used birth weight as the primary factor in diagnosing a particular case as premature. Although there is a very high correlation between birth weight and estimated gestational age, it is clear that low birth weight does not always indicate a preterm birth.

Our focus in this chapter is on the psychological sequelae of the *preterm* birth, that is, on infants born before 37 weeks of gestation have been completed (American Academy of Pediatrics, 1967). In order to have uniform terminology, we will use the word preterm to describe studies in which the authors have defined "prematurity" by the standard of birth weight.

The incidence of preterm births varies widely around the world, and it also varies according to subpopulations within the United States (Ritz, 1975). Available statistics suggest that preterm births occur in 7-12% of births in the United States, with the incidence being higher for nonwhites than for whites (Hellman & Pritchard, 1971; Ritz, 1975; Speert, 1971; Taylor, 1976).

The preterm baby is faced with a higher probability of developing a variety of medical complications, including hyaline membrane disease, infection, intracranial hemorrhage, and central nervous system damage (Hellman & Pritchard, 1971; Korones, Lancaster, & Roberts, 1972; Ritz, 1975; Speert, 1971). Preterm births are also the leading cause of neonatal death (Hellman & Pritchard, 1971; Lesser, 1973; Taylor, 1976). The average mortality rate is around 20% and the mortality rate climbs as gestational age and birth weight decline (Speert, 1971; Stewart & Reynolds, 1974). Preterm infants clearly look different on a wide variety of measures, including skin color, skin texture, and plantar creases, and may exhibit a series of distinctive neurological signs, etc. (Hellman & Pritchard, 1971; Korones, Lancaster, & Roberts, 1972; Ritz, 1975).

For the parent the preterm birth is an unexpected event. Although labor is expected in the future, the beginning of labor at a point in time well ahead of the predicted date is an occurrence for which parents are unprepared. Six to eight weeks of preparation time is lost, both in terms of psychological preparation and in terms of practical preparation for the new infant. The atmosphere in the hospital will probably be more similar to that surrounding a medical emergency than is the atmosphere for the average birth (Owens, 1960).

The infant is born earlier and more unexpectedly than a term baby, the medical atmosphere may be quite intimidating, the child behaves differently and looks different from term infants, and the parents face a much higher probability that the baby is seriously ill or even dying. What are the psychological consequences for the parents? Our focus now will be on research that has attempted to answer this question.

## PARENTAL REACTIONS

Although we have titled this section parental reactions, most of the available data pertain to the mother's reaction to the preterm birth. Little systematic information is currently available on the father's reaction.

### Parent-Infant Interaction

As Minde, Ford, Celhoffer, and Boukydis (1975) have pointed out, mothers differ in their interactions with the preterm infant. However, available evidence suggests that as a group, mothers of normal infants may exhibit patterns of interacting with their newborn infants different from those exhibited by mothers of preterm infants.

Mothers of full-term infants appear to hold their babies closer to their bodies and to smile at them more than do mothers of preterm infants. Leifer, Leiderman, Barnett, and Williams (1972) observed such differences when comparing three groups of mothers. One group of mothers was separated from their newborn preterm infants for periods of 3–12 weeks; the mothers were allowed to see their infants but were not allowed to hold, cuddle, or handle them. The second group of mothers, who also had preterm infants, was allowed (after the first two or three days) to enter the nursery, handle the baby, and assist in caretaking. The third group was made up of mothers who had term infants; these mothers were also allowed full contact with their infants during feeding periods, four or five times a day. The most consistently observed findings were differences between mothers of full-term infants and mothers of preterm infants. Mothers of full-term infants tended to hold the baby close to them more frequently than did mothers of preterm infants, and mothers of full-term infants smiled at their babies more often than did mothers of preterm babies.

An intriguing serendipitous finding of the Leifer et al. (1972) study was that six instances of divorce occurred in the group of mothers who had not been allowed to interact freely with their infants. Two mothers out of the total sample relinquished custody of their infants; both of these women were in the separated group.

Seashore, Leifer, Barnett, and Leiderman (1973) provided further information on interaction patterns of preterm infants and their mothers. Maternal self-confidence appeared related to early separation from the preterm infant for primiparas. In this study, two groups of mother-infant pairs were used to investigate the effects of mother-infant separation on maternal self-confidence. One group of mothers had preterm infants, and they were permitted only to view their infants during the time the infants were in intensive care, a period of 3–12 weeks. The other group was also composed of preterm infants and their mothers, but these mothers were allowed to enter the intensive care nursery and handle, diaper, and assist in the feeding of the infant. Results indicated that being allowed to interact with the infant did not by itself produce a difference in the mother's self-confidence either in interacting socially with or in taking care of the infant. However, mother-infant separation did have a differential impact on the mother, depending on whether or not she was a primipara. Whereas separation did not affect the degree of self-confidence for multiparas, separation did significantly affect self-confidence in primiparas. Of the mothers of preterm infants who were primiparas, those who were permitted contact with the infant had a significantly higher level of confidence about interacting with the baby than did the mothers of preterm infants who were permitted only visual contact with the newborn.

Evidence suggests that the behavior of mothers of preterm infants differs from that of mothers of full-term infants in other ways. Crawford (1977) compared mothers of preterm infants, with an average gestational age of 28.3 weeks at birth, with mothers of full-term infants, who averaged 39.7 weeks at birth. The infants and their mothers were observed at home when the infants were six and eight months old. The most consistently observed difference between the preterm and the full-term infant-mother pairs was in the amount of time the mothers spent in looking after the infant's needs. Mothers of preterm infants spent a greater portion of their time feeding, cleaning and diapering their infants than did mothers of full-term infants.

Additional findings suggest that mothers of preterm infants show less emotional involvement with their infants than do mothers of full-term babies. In a comparison of mothers of preterm infants and mothers of full-term infants, Brown and Bakeman (1977) observed a group of inner-city, low-income, black mother-infant pairs. Twenty-six preterm infants, with a mean gestational age of 32 weeks, and 23 full-term infants, with a mean gestational age of 40 weeks, were studied. A social worker visited the home and recorded ratings of the "emotional and verbal responsivity of the mother" toward her infant nine months after discharge from the hospital. Results indicated that mothers of preterm infants were likely to show less emotional involvement with their infants than were mothers of full-term infants.

## Emotional Reactions

Common sense, as well as clinical observation, has indicated for some time that the emotional response of parents to the birth of a preterm infant is different from the reaction to the birth of a full-term infant. The notion has been that a preterm birth represents a significantly more stressful and unpleasant situation for the parents than does a full-term birth.

The suggestion has been made that the mothers of preterm infants are likely to experience a significant degree of anxiety and guilt, such as anxiety about the child, its size, chance of survival, and caretaking activities. The mother also may experience guilt about whether or not she precipitated the child's premature birth, along with guilt because the nurse is more competent in caring for the child than she is (Prugh, 1953). Johnson and Grubbs (1975) have suggested that the mother's expectations and beliefs about how the baby will behave are based on information about full-term babies. Because the preterm infant differs in looks and behavior from expectations, the mother may feel uncomfortable and inadequate interacting with her infant.

Further data suggest that mothers of preterm infants view their pregnancies more negatively than do mothers of full-term infants. Although not directly investigating the consequences of preterm birth, Blau, Slaff and Easton, (1963) reported some interesting differences between the mothers of preterm and full-term infants in their recollections about the pregnancy. Blau et al. conducted extensive interviews with the mothers of a group of preterm infants and a matched group of mothers of full-term infants. Interviewers administered a wide variety of personality measures, including such tests as the Rorschach, the Thematic Apperception Test, and the Wechsler intelligence test, one to two days postpartum. Based on the data gathered on each of the women, ratings were made of her on a variety of scales, including some designed to measure her attitude toward the pregnancy. Results indicated that mothers of preterm infants had significantly more negative attitudes toward their pregnancies than did mothers of full-term infants.

Another investigation of the psychological impact of preterm birth focused on mothers who had at least two children, one of whom was born preterm and one of whom was born full-term (Bidder, Crowe, & Gray, 1974). When the preterm children were 2.8–3.5 years the mothers were asked to rate, on semantic differential scales, the preterm child, the full-term child, and the "ideal child." The mothers were also asked about their experiences with the pregnancies and births. Results indicated no reliable differences in the semantic differential ratings of the preterm and full-term children. However, the mothers reported being more anxious in the hospital and being more anxious at home after the birth of the preterm infant than after the birth of the full-term infant.

Both the study conducted by Blau et al. (1963) and the study conducted by Bidder et al. (1974) suggested that mothers of preterm infants differ from mothers of full-term infants in their recollections about the pregnancy and the immediate postpartum period. It is the study published in 1960 by Kaplan and Mason, however, that is probably the most often cited confirmation of the view that the mother of the preterm infant faces a significant crisis. Because it is cited so frequently, we will examine the Kaplan and Mason study in more detail.

The report of Kaplan and Mason was based on a sample of 60 families who were interviewed during the period after the birth. Information obtained from these interviews was examined and several conclusions drawn. The authors indicated that for the preterm infant labor and delivery took place in an atmosphere that had more of the characteristics of a medical emergency than of a term birth. The preterm birth was unexpected for the mother, and after delivery the mother had a greater concern about the baby. On first observing the infant in the nursery, many of the mothers were frightened by the baby's appearance. Reviewing these observations, Kaplan and Mason then enumerated a series of "psychological tasks" that mothers of preterm infants must complete in order to resolve the crisis of the preterm birth.

Kaplan and Mason hypothesized four such tasks. The first is the preparation for the possible death of the infant. The second task involves the recognition by the mother that she has failed to produce a full-term infant. The third task is the formation of a normal maternal attachment as the baby shows improvement. The fourth task involves preparing to care for the baby by reading, obtaining appropriate information from the physician and the nurse, and discussing the situation with other mothers.

Kaplan and Mason hypothesized that for the mother to deal successfully with preterm birth, she must complete each of the four proposed psychological tasks. If the mother fails in these tasks, then psychopathological patterns of varying degrees of severity can be expected.

Kaplan and Mason's ideas have been included frequently in nursing and medical texts without a significant degree of critical evaluation. In a subsequent section we will examine the positive and negative features of the group of studies that we are reviewing. It should be noted at this point, however, that in spite of the important contribution made by the Kaplan and Mason (1960) report, the study did not include a control group and the description of the results was not complete enough for an assessment of the appropriateness of the four proposed psychological tasks.

Evidence does exist indicating greater emotional distress during the early postpartum period in mothers of preterm, versus mothers of full-term, infants. Choi (1973) interviewed the mothers of 20 preterm infants (defined by a birth weight of 2500 grams or less) and a matched group of mothers of full-term infants. Three to five days postpartum the mothers were interviewed, using a questionnaire that contained items designed to assess the degree of anxiety and depression experienced by the women. The mothers of preterm infants obtained significantly higher scores on the questionnaire, indicating a higher degree of anxiety and depression. Highly reliable correlations were also found between the infant's birthweight and the mother's anxiety-depression score and between the infant's gestational age and the anxiety-depression score of the mother. As birth weight and gestational age decreased, the mother's anxiety-depression increased. Not only were the mothers of preterm infants significantly more anxious and depressed during the early postpartum period, but the degree of depression-anxiety was significantly related to the birth weight and gestational age of the child.

The presence of problems with self-esteem in a group of preterm mothers was reported by Cramer (1976). Thirteen mothers were given a semistructured interview after they delivered preterm infants. No control group was interviewed, and the description of the methodology employed was less than detailed, but Cramer reported some interesting conclusions. These mothers of preterm infants were reported frequently to experience feelings of failure. Although not all had obvious self-esteem difficulties, almost all were reported to have feelings of guilt. The mothers also indicated that when their infants were taken away for medical care, they experienced an emotional void; the separation also heightened their feelings of failure. Cramer concluded that the data indicated that the birth of a preterm infant was in fact a severe psychological crisis for the mothers.

The days and weeks after the preterm delivery are times of emotional crisis for the parents, and there may be differences in parenting style that can be noted as late as eight years after the birth of the child (Blake, Stewart, & Turcan, 1975). One hundred and sixty infants weighing 1500 grams or less, and their parents, were observed over an eight-year period by Blake et al. In the first six months mothers were reported to go through three phases: the first, a "honeymoon" phase in which excitement prevailed; the second, a period of exhaustion in which the mother complained of a series of problems with feeding, caring for the infant, etc.; the third phase, in which the problems of phase two disappeared and the mother interacted with her child with confidence. These researchers also reported that the parents of preterm infants continue to need much reassurance as the child grows, although it is possible that parents of full-term infants also want considerable reassurance from physicians. Bidder et al. (1974) indicated that there is also a tendency for the parents of low birth weight infants to be somewhat overprotective toward these children in the child's early years.

Blake and associates (1975) indicated that fathers tended to express anxieties quite similar to those expressed by the mothers of low birth weight infants. The fathers were reported to be well involved with their infants. The authors even speculated that a possible advantage of low birth weight may be the increased probability of more paternal involvement with the child.

Up to this point, the research we have reviewed has generally indicated a reliable difference between the parents of preterm infants and the parents of full-term infants. Not all available data, however, indicate such a difference. A notable exception to the previously reviewed material is the study reported by Smith, Schwartz, Mandell, Siberstein, Dalack, and Sacks (1969).

Smith et al. (1969) reported the results of a study of 36 preterm mothers and a matched group of 33 full-term mothers. The mothers were interviewed three to five days postpartum, and the focus of the interview was on their feelings about pregnancy and their reactions to the newborn infant. The interviewers rated the mother's mood, her degree of acceptance of the mothering role, and her concern for the baby's welfare. Results indicated no reliable differences between the mothers of preterm infants and the mothers of full-term infants on any of the ratings. It should be noted, however, that the ratings of the mothers' reactions were in the direction we would expect from the research we have reviewed here; i.e., preterm mothers did have a higher mean rating of depression, which failed to reach traditional levels of significance.

Bidder et al. (1974) asked mothers who had both a preterm infant and a full-term infant to give semantic differential ratings to both infants. These researchers failed to find any difference between the ratings.

Although preterm births are a relatively frequent occurrence, the volume of research on the psychological consequences for the parents is still relatively restricted. Not only is the sheer volume of research rather small, but the research also suffers from methodological shortcomings. One problem has been a failure of some research projects to include an appropriate control group; such a failure, although understandable on practical grounds, makes it impossible to draw conclusions about the possible effects of the preterm birth itself. As we see in Chapter 4, term birth can produce a variety of unpleasant emotional reactions in the mother, and it is only by including an appropriate control group that firm conclusions can be drawn about the unique impact of a preterm birth.

As we indicated in the beginning of this chapter, the area of research has been plagued by a lack of reliable nomenclature. *Preterm* and *premature* have been defined most often on the basis of birth weight; current practice is moving in the desirable direction of specifying both birth weight and estimated gestational age. Although there is a very high and reliable correlation between estimated gestational age and birth weight, discrepancies do exist. Therefore, it is impossible to differentiate the possible effects of preterm birth from those of low birth weight.

Another problematic factor in the available research involves the dependent variables used to assess parental psychological reactions. Parental reactions have not been measured consistently. Most often, researchers have developed their own rating scales specifically for their investigation of preterm birth. Although the reliabilities reported are usually quite good, the diversity of measures makes it difficult to compare results obtained in different studies. Future projects could profitably include established methods of assessment in conjunction with those developed for a particular investigation.

Now that we have indicated certain possible limitations of these studies, we shall proceed to draw some generalizations from the currently available data. It should be clear, however, that such generalizations must be regarded with a degree of caution since the research projects on which they are based often have suffered from methodological limitations.

What do the data suggest about the reactions of parents to the preterm birth of an infant? Do the data in fact lend support to the hypothesis that the preterm birth is a significantly greater crisis than a full-term birth? Our conclusion here is a tentative yes.

The available data suggest that the birth of a preterm infant represents a crisis for the parents. Mothers of preterm infants appear to experience a significantly higher degree of psychological discomfort postpartum than do mothers of full-term infants. The preterm birth is characterized by anxiety on the part of the mother (Bidder, Crowe, & Gray, 1974; Blake, Steward, & Turcan, 1975; Choi, 1973; Cramer, 1976; Kaplan & Mason, 1960). Although the lack of control groups in some studies restricts our confidence in the generalization, the findings from those studies that included a comparison group of term mothers indicate that the mothers of preterm infants tend to experience more anxiety in the postpartum period.

The possibility that guilt and depression occur more frequently in mothers of preterm infants is suggested by the data, but the conclusion must be considerably more tentative than that about anxiety. Although this position is clearly congruent with common sense and clinical expectation, the available data can be regarded as only suggesting that mothers of preterm infants feel more depression and guilt than do mothers of full-term infants (Choi, 1973; Cramer, 1976) in the puerperium.

Greater involvement of the father with preterm as compared to full-term infants could represent a positive consequence of such births. According to Blake et al. (1975), this possibility requires further empirical evaluation.

(Although beyond the scope of our present review, another potential consequence of the preterm birth should be noted. Some data suggest that there is a reliable relationship between being a preterm or low birthweight infant and subsequently being physically abused by a parent [e.g., Fomufod, 1976; Stern, 1973]. The precise causal relationships are still unclear, but the evidence suggests that the relationship between condition of birth and later child abuse exists. For further discussion of this matter, the reader is referred to Parke and Collmer [1975].)

## THE CRISIS OF THE PRETERM BIRTH: CONCEPTUALIZING OUTCOME

Our review of the current research has suggested that the birth of a preterm infant represents a crisis for the parents, and the indications are that parents experience a significantly greater degree of psychological distress following the birth of a preterm infant than they do following the birth of a full-term infant. In this section we will examine a conceptual framework proposed for understanding the crisis of the preterm birth and examine some of the variables that have been suggested as predictive of a good outcome of that crisis.

The birth of a preterm infant is a crisis. This event produces a significant disruption for the parents. Crisis theory provides a good framework for conceptualizing the problems faced by the parents of the preterm infant (Calhoun, Selby, & King, 1976; Caplan, 1960, 1964).

As Caplan and his co-workers have suggested, the conceptualizaton of the psychological reactions of a parent to the birth of a preterm infant should take three dimensions into account: cognitive reactions, affective reactions, and interaction of the parent with available resources.

*Cognitive reactions* in this context refer to the parent's general understanding of the situation, especially the search for information directly relevant to the preterm birth. It has been suggested that in order to increase the probability of a successful psychological outcome, the parent should seek out and assimilate reliable information on the causes of the preterm birth and the possible consequences for the infant. The psychodynamic perspective suggests that attention be given to possible cognitive distortions by the parent, such as denial or avoidance of accurate information about the baby's condition.

The *affective reactions* important in the crisis of the preterm birth are the negative feelings that parents experience. This dimension has been the most often studied. Anxiety is one predominant response pattern, and we have also noted that some investigators have reported depressive and guilt reactions. The important factor here seems to be for the parent to verbalize negative feelings that are appropriate to the degree of situational stress. The psychodynamic perspective suggests that defense mechanisms such as denial and suppression of negative feelings be recognized since extreme reliance on these may lead to a poor resolution of the crisis.

*Resources* are anything that can be helpful to the individual in a crisis situation. For the parents of the preterm infant, important resources include each other, relatives, friends, physicians, and nurses. A crucial factor in the resolution of any crisis is putting the individual in contact with the appropriate resources. Preterm births are no exception. The parents should be supported in their attempts to seek help from resources available to them.

Using these three categories of information as guidelines, we will now consider some practical issues in working with the parents of preterm infants. We do not intend this as a complete description of all factors that must be considered in assisting the parents since such reviews are available elsewhere (Kennell & Klaus, 1971; Klaus & Kennell, 1976; Korones, Lancaster, & Roberts, 1972). Our goal is to consider factors that may be important in dealing with the psychological issues faced by the parents of preterm infants.

Awareness of the type of reaction that the parents are experiencing is important. The data presented here give a general picture of what happens in the average case. Although the present information should be useful as a frame of reference, the psychological truism about every case being different applies here as well. It is important to try to obtain an understanding of the psychological responses of each individual since the specific intervention indicated will vary from case to case.

The framework given above should be useful in organizing information about the reactions of specific parents. Does the parent have a reasonably accurate cognitive grasp of the situation and is the parent actively engaging in information seeking? To the extent that the parent is actively seeking information and indicates a generally accurate understanding of the present situation, a better psychological outcome can be expected than if these conditions are not being met (Caplan & Mason, 1965; Mason, 1964). Caregivers (e.g., nurses, physicians, social workers, and psychologists) may be able to encourage the seeking of accurate information or to provide such information directly. Health care personnel should be aware of the cognitive reactions of the parents, being particularly concerned where there is no active seeking of information or where there is a distortion of the actual situation.

In attending to the parent's affective reaction to the preterm birth, a clear danger signal may be the absence of negative feelings. For example, mothers who verbalize no anxiety about the infant and who express no depression or concern in the situation may be providing a danger signal. A very persistent rule in clinical folklore suggests that individuals with high levels of affective reaction tend to show improvement from psychiatric problems to a greater degree than do those who do not show response. A modified version of this rule seems to apply to preterm births. Mothers who have a moderate to high level of anxiety probably will have a better outcome to the crisis of the preterm birth than will mothers who verbalize little or no anxiety. Where the mother shows little or no anxiety, referral to an appropriate mental health professional (psychiatrist, psychologist, or social worker) may be appropriate.

A general assessment of the individual's resources and an assessment of the interaction of the individual with those resources may also prove useful. To what extent are relatives, friends, physicians, neighbors, public health nurses, etc., available and willing to assist the parents of the preterm infant? As a rough rule of thumb, we would suggest that the more resources available, the better the chance of a successful outcome for the parent. Resources that are supportive and understanding can be very useful in helping the parent understand the situation accurately and verbalize appropriate feelings about the preterm birth (Caplan, 1960; Caplan & Mason,

1965). An exception to the usefulness of resources, however, is the situation in which relatives, friends, etc., discourage the parent from seeking accurate information and from accurately conceptualizing the situation and encourage the parent to verbalize feelings inappropriate to the situation. Not only is an understanding of the sheer number of resources important, but an understanding of the quality of that support also is important.

Available evidence and theorizing suggest that health care personnel should do their best to arrange the hospital situation so as to minimize or even eliminate the separation of parents and preterm infants (Klaus & Kennell, 1976; Leifer et al., 1972; Seashore et al., 1973). Although separation is probably never desirable, it may be particularly distressing for primiparas. The psychological impact of mother-infant separation is probably never good, and separation may be particularly a problem for the mother giving birth to her first child.

In a variety of subareas of psychiatry and psychology, there has recently been great interest in the antecedents and consequences of the types of causes that observers ascribe to certain events (e.g., Calhoun, Peirce, Walters, & Dawes, 1974; Calhoun, Selby, & Wroten, 1977; Selby & Calhoun, 1975; Jones et al., 1972; King et al., 1978). Naive observers develop causal explanations for behaviors that may not necessarily agree with the explanations advanced by experts in a certain area (Calhoun, Johnson, & Boardman, 1975; Johnson, Calhoun, & Boardman, 1975). Available evidence suggests that mothers of preterm infants also tend to develop a variety of causal "explanations" for the preterm birth of the infant that may not be congruent with accepted medical explanations (or absence of explanation) of a particular case. Cramer (1976), for example, in his interviews of mothers after a preterm birth, indicated that some of the explanations for the preterm birth given by the mothers included too much sexual activity, feeling inadequate, and enjoying her job. Since the cause ascribed to a particular behavior may have consequences for the subsequent psychological functioning of the individual (Calhoun, Selby, & Wroten, 1977; Jones et al., 1972), attending health care personnel should become familiar with the types of explanations given by parents for the preterm birth of their infant. Whenever possible, the physician or nurse should provide a concise and clear medical explanation of the cause of the birth. If a medical explanation does not present itself, then the attending medical personnel may provide a reasonable hypothesis based on the available data in the case.

Finally, we would like to suggest that it is highly important that the attending medical personnel take sufficient time to explain and answer any questions that the parents may have about the preterm birth or the preterm infant. As noted previously, having a good understanding of a problem situation is an important asset in overcoming a crisis. The medical personnel working with parents throughout the pregnancy, delivery, and the postpartum period are in a position to provide such information as well as emotional support and reassurance.

## REFERENCES


American Academy of Pediatrics. Nomenclature for duration of gestation, birth weight, and intra-uterine growth. *Pediatrics,* 1967, *39,* 935.

BARNETT, C. R., LEIDERMAN, P. H., GROBSTEIN, R., and KLAUS, M. Neonatal separation: the maternal side of interactional deprivation. *Pediatrics,* 1970, *45,* 197-205.

BIDDER, R. T., CROWE, E. A., and GRAY, O. P. Mothers' attitudes to preterm infants. *Archives of Disease in Childhood,* 1974, *49,* 766-770.

BLAKE, A., STEWART, A., and TURCAN, D. Parents of babies of very low birth weight. *CIBA Foundation Symposium,* 1975, *33,* 271-288.

BLAU, A., SLAFF, B., and EASTON, K. The psychogenic etiology of premature births. *Psychosomatic Medicine,* 1963, *25,* 201-211.

BROWN, J. V., and BAKEMAN, R. Antecedents of emotional involvement in mothers of premature and fullterm infants. Paper presented to the Society for Research in Child Development, New Orleans, 1977.

CALHOUN, L. G., JOHNSON, R. E., and BOARDMAN, W. K. Attribution of depression to internal-external and stable-unstable causes. *Psychological Reports,* 1975, *36,* 463-466.

CALHOUN, L. G., PEIRCE, J. R., WALTERS, S., and DAWES, A. S. Determinants of social rejection for help-seeking. *Journal of Consulting and Clinical Psychology,* 1974, *42,* 618.

CALHOUN, L. G., SELBY, J. W., and KING, H. E. *Dealing with crisis.* Englewood Cliffs: Prentice-Hall, 1976.

CALHOUN, L. G., SELBY, J. W., and WROTEN, J. Situational constraint and type of causal explanation. *Journal of Research in Personality,* 1977, *11,* 95-100.

CAPLAN, G. Patterns of parental response to the crisis of premature birth. *Psychiatry,* 1960, *23,* 365-374.

———. *Principles of preventive psychiatry.* New York: Basic Books, 1964.

CAPLAN, G., and MASON, E. H. Four studies of crisis in parents of prematures. *Community Mental Health Journal,* 1965, *1,* 149-161.

CHOI, M. W. A comparison of maternal psychological reactions to premature and full-size newborns. *Maternal-Child Nursing Journal,* 1973, *2,* 1-13.

COHLER, B. J., WEISS, J. L., and GRUNEBAU, H. U. Child-care attitudes and emotional disturbance among mothers of young children. *Genetic Psychology Monographs,* 1970, *82,* 3-48.

COREY, E. J., MILLER, C. L., and WIDLAK, F. W. Factors contributing to child abuse. *Nursing Research,* 1975, *24,* 293-295.

CRAMER, B. A mother's reactions to the birth of a premature baby. In M. H. Klaus and J. H. Kennell *Maternal-infant bonding.* Saint Louis: Mosby, 1976.

CRAWFORD, J. W. The premature infant and mother-infant interaction: a preliminary report. Paper presented to the Society for Research in Child Development, New Orleans, 1977.

CROPLEY, C., and BLOOM, R. S. An interaction guide for a neonatal special-care unit. *Pediatrics,* 1975, *55,* 287-290.

ELMER, E., and GREGG, G. S. Developmental characteristics of abused children. *Pediatrics,* 1967, *40,* 596-602.

Fanaroff, A. A., Kennell, J. H., and Klaus, M. H. Follow-up of low birth weight infants: the predictive value of maternal visiting patterns. *Pediatrics,* 1972, *49,* 287–290.

Fomufod, A. K. Low birth weight and early neonatal separation as factors in child abuse. *Journal of the National Medical Association,* 1976, *17,* 106–109.

Gruenwald, P. Letter: not all small neonates are premature. *American Journal of Public Health,* 1974, *64,* 1102.

Hellman, L. M., and Pritchard, J. A. *Williams Obstetrics* (14th ed.). New York: Appleton-Century-Crofts, 1971.

Iffy, L. Diagnosis of fetal maturity. In R. M. Wynn (ed.), *Obstetrics and gynecology annual,* vol. 2. New York: Appleton-Century-Crofts, 1973.

Johnson, R. E., Calhoun, L. G., and Boardman, W. K. The effect of severity, consistency, and typicalness information on clinicians' causal attributions. *Journal of Clinical Psychology,* 1975, *31,* 600–604.

Johnson, S. H., and Grubbs, J. P. The premature infant's reflex behaviors. *JOGN Nursing,* 1975, *4,* 15–20.

Jones, E. E., Kanouse, D. E., et al *Attribution: perceiving the causes of behavior.* Morristown: General Learning Press, 1972.

Kaplan, D. M., and Mason, E. A. Maternal reaction to premature birth viewed as an acute emotional disorder. *American Journal of Orthopsychiatry,* 1960, *30,* 539–552.

Kenell, J. H., and Klaus, M. H. Care of the mother of the high-risk infant. *Clinical Obstetrics and Gynecology,* 1971, *14,* 926–954.

King, H. E., Rotter, M., Calhoun, L. G., and Selby, J. W. Perceptions of the rape incident. *Journal of Community Psychology,* 1978, *6,* 74–77.

Klaus, M. H., Jerrauld, R., Kreger, N., and McAlpine, W. Maternal attachment. *New England Journal of Medicine,* 1972, *286,* 460–463.

Klaus, M. H., and Kennell, J. H. *Maternal-infant bonding.* St. Louis: Mosby, 1976.

Korones, S. B., Lancaster, J., and Roberts, F. B. *High risk newborn infants.* St. Louis: Mosby, 1972.

Leifer, A. D., Leiderman, P. H., Barnett, C. R., and Williams, J. A. Effects of mother-infant separation on maternal attachment behavior. *Child Development,* 1972, *43,* 1203–1218.

Lesser, A. Trends in maternal and child care. In M. H. Wallace, E. M. Gold, and E. Luis (eds.), *Maternal and child health practices.* Springfield: Charles C Thomas, 1973.

Mason, E. A. A method for predicting crisis outcome for mothers of premature babies. *Briefs,* 1964, *28,* 36–39.

McFarland, M. B., and Reinhart, J. B. The development of motherliness. *Children,* 1959, *6,* 48.

Minde, K., Ford, L., Celhoffer, L., and Boukydis, C. Interactions of mothers and nurses with premature infants. *Canadian Medical Journal,* 1975, *113,* 741–745.

Osofsky, J. D., and Danzger, B. Relationship between neonatal characteristics and mother-infant interaction. *Developmental Psychology,* 1974, *10,* 124–130.

Owens, C. Parents' response to premature birth. *American Journal of Nursing,* 1960, *60,* 1113–1118.

Parke, R. D., and Collmer, C. W. Child abuse: an interdisciplinary analysis. In E. M. Hetherington (ed.), *Child development research.* Chicago: University of Chicago Press, 1975.

Paton, J. B., and Fisher, D. E. Dysmaturity. In R. M. Wynn (ed.), *Obstetrics and gynecology annual,* vol. 2. New York: Appleton-Century-Crofts, 1973.

PRUGH, D. G. Emotional problems of the premature infant's parents. *Nursing Outlook,* 1953, *1,* 461-464.

RITZ, A. The preterm infant. In E. J. Dickason and M. O. Schult (eds.), *Maternal and infant care.* New York: McGraw-Hill, 1975.

SCIPIEN, G. M., BARNARD, M. U., CHARD, M. A., HOWE, J., and PHILLIPS, P. J. *Comprehensive pediatric nursing.* New York: McGraw-Hill, 1975.

SEASHORE, M. J., LEIFER, A. D., BARNETT, C. R., and LEIDERMAN, P. H. The effects of denial of early mother-infant interaction on maternal self-confidence. *Journal of Personality and Social Psychology,* 1973, *26,* 369–378.

SELBY, J. W., and CALHOUN, L. G. Social perception of suicide. *Journal of Consulting and Clinical Psychology,* 1975, *43,* 431.

SMITH, N., SCHWARTZ, J. R., MANDELL, W., SIBERSTEIN, R. M., DALACK, J. D., and SACKS, S. Mothers' psychological reactions to premature and full-size newborns. *Archives of General Psychiatry,* 1969, *21,* 177–181.

SOLNIT, A. J., and STARK, N. H. Mourning and the birth of a defective child. *Psychoanalytic Study of the Child,* 1961, *16,* 523–537.

SPEERT, H. Premature labor. In D. N. Danforth (ed.), *Textbook of obstetrics and gynecology* (2d ed.). New York: Harper & Row, 1971.

STERN, L. Premature separation of infant and mother may be a factor in child abuse. *Hospital Practice,* 1973, *8,* 117–123.

STEWART, A. L., & REYNOLDS, E. R. Improved prognosis for infants of very low birth weight. *Pediatrics,* 1974, *54,* 724–735.

TAYLOR, E. S. *Beck's obstetrical practice and fetal medicine* (10th ed.). Baltimore: Williams & Wilkins, 1976.

WIENER, G. Psychological correlates of premature birth: a review. *Journal of Nervous and Mental Disease,* 1962, *134,* 129–144.

WORTIS, H. Discussion of Kaplan-Mason study. *American Journal of Orthopsychiatry,* 1960, *30,* 547-552.

# Chapter 6

# The Psychological Impact of Having a Handicapped Baby

IT IS ESTIMATED THAT an infant with a significant birth defect is born every two minutes in the United States. This means 250,000 children with birth defects are born annually in this country—1 out of every 16 babies (Apgar & Beck, 1974). It is unlikely that anyone is ever adequately prepared to be the parent of a handicapped child.

Parenthood has been described as an opportunity for enriching one's own identity and affirming one's generativity and as an opportunity to pass on one's ideals and values (Meadow & Meadow, 1971). Persons who have been socialized to this conception of parenthood face a different socialization process when they become parents of a handicapped child. Two special tasks have been described for parents of handicapped children: learning to cope with feelings of grief and sorrow and learning to meet effectively the special needs of the child (Meadow & Meadow, 1971).

This chapter will focus on the initial parental response to the new role of being the parent of a handicapped baby. Research on the following issues will be reviewed: the emotional reaction of parents to the birth of a handicapped baby; early parenting responses; variables that affect the response of parents; how the diagnosis is communicated to parents; and how parents wish they had been told. The research on these topics will be evaluated, and suggestions will be offered to professionals for effective support of parents of handicapped babies.

## EMOTIONAL REACTIONS TO THE BIRTH OF A HANDICAPPED CHILD

Parental reaction to the birth of a handicapped baby has been likened to the emotional crisis following the death of a child in that the parent must mourn the loss of the expected normal infant. In addition, the parent must become attached to the actual, living damaged child (Solnit & Stark, 1961). Two recent studies have explored parents' initial reactions to the birth of a child with congenital anomalies within the framework of this theory of grief and mourning.

Interviews with 22 mothers of babies with birth defects were conducted by Kennedy (1970). A broad range of birth defects, from mild to major, was included. The purpose of the study was to investigate whether the reactions of mothers fell into the time limited sequence that is associated with grief reactions. Three clinical interviews were held with the mothers, with the initial interview taking place in the period 7–24 days after the birth of the child and later interviews occurring in the next weeks and months.

Some focus was built into the interviews: the mothers were aware that they had been selected because they were parents of handicapped babies, and the interviewer asked clarifying questions to elicit further comments about feelings. For the most part, however, the mothers were given the opportunity to discuss freely their feelings following the birth of the handicapped baby. The interviews were recorded for later analysis, and notations were made about body language during the interviews.

In analyzing the data collected in the clinical interviews, Kennedy (1970) looked for behavior and statements of affect that could be related to the grief process. These were described as follows:

1. Protest. Shock, numbness, disbelief, anger.
2. Despair, Disappointment, loss, hopelessness, physical symptoms such as insomnia and lack of appetite.
3. Guilt. The mother blames herself or seems preoccupied with thoughts about actions she took during pregnancy that may have caused the baby's defect.
4. Recall of prebirth longings for the idealized infant. The mother tells how during pregnancy she thought about how she would have a boy or a girl, and she mentions the names she and her husband selected.
5. Cathexis of the defective baby. Emotional significance of the baby is evidenced by referring to the baby by its given name.

Each interview was analyzed for the presence or absence of the above behaviors or statements and a rating was made of whether the behavior was mild or strong. The reliability of the ratings was checked by an independent judge; reliability coefficients were relatively low, ranging from .35 to .54.

The findings from this analysis suggested that the mothers of handicapped newborns experienced a process of mourning that was time limited and characterized by behaviors specific for each phase. Between one and four weeks after delivery, evidence of protest and despair were present. Attachment to the baby became increasingly evident in the four weeks to two months after birth.

The attachment process, following grief and mourning, was further explored by Drotar, Baskiewicz, Irvin, Kennell, and Klaus (1975). The parents (20 mothers and 5 fathers) of 20 children with congenital malformations were interviewed regarding their reactions to the births. The children exhibited a range of congenital malformations including Down's syndrome, cleft palate and lip, microcephaly, absence of forearm, encephalocele, and mental retardation of unknown etiology. The interview information was obtained by a series of open-ended questions regarding parents' emotional reactions and perceptions of the child's malformations. The interviews, which were taped, took approximately one and a half hours; the scheduling of the interviews ranged from within a few days of the birth to as long as five years later. Sixty-five percent of the interviews were held within the first year. Analysis of each interview involved transcription followed by an analysis of statements made in the interview. The analyses were made by two researchers who did not conduct the initial interviews or have information concerning the children's problems.

The structured interview involved five kinds of question:

1. Parental perception of the child's deformity. When did you first suspect your baby had a problem? How did you find out?
2. Parental feelings. What has happened since then up to the present time with your baby? With the both of you?
3. Assessment of parental attachment. Does it seem like the baby is yours? Do you feel close to the baby? How did you go about naming the baby?
4. Effects of the anomaly. Have you shared your feelings together? Do you find yourself blue? Angry? Irritable? What is your outlook for the future? Could you compare your family life since the baby was born with the way it was before?
5. Parental attitudes toward handling the situation. What helped? What didn't help? What suggestions would you have for other families in the same situation?

Despite the great variation in the children's malformations and in parental backgrounds, a number of common themes emerged in these interviews. In general, the parents vividly recalled the events surrounding the birth and described both their reactions and the reactions of others around them in great detail. Looking at these common themes, Drotar et al. (1975) constructed a hypothetical model to summarize the complex reactions of the parents. This sequence reflects the course of the reactions of most parents in this study to the birth of their congenitally malformed infant:

1. Shock. All but one mother reported that they had expected a normal child. They reported initial feelings of overwhelming shock, periods of crying, and feelings of helplessness.

2. Denial. Parents reported a wish to be free from the situation or to deny its impact. Although every parent reported his or her disbelief, the intensity of the denial varied considerably, depending on the visibility of the malformation.

3. Sadness, anger, anxiety. Twelve parents described their sadness and noted that they cried a great deal. Seven families were disrupted by angry feelings directed toward themselves, toward the child, or outwardly toward the hospital staff or other people. Eleven parents described intense feelings of anxiety, particularly related to fears that the baby would die. Hesitance regarding attachment to the baby was seen in almost all the mothers.

4. Adaptation. Ten of the parents reported a gradual lessening of the anxiety and intense emotional reactions. As feelings of emotional upset lessened, they reported increased comfort with their situation and confidence in their ability to start caring for the babies. Parents varied in the length of time required to reach the period of adaptation. In many cases the adaptation seemed to be incomplete; one parent reported that "tears come even yet, years after the baby's birth" (p. 713).

5. Reorganization. This was a complex time in which parents described a more rewarding type of interaction with their infants. Parents dealt with possible causes for the defect or learned to assure themselves that the baby's problem was "nothing I'd done." Parents' mutual support was emphasized as crucial. Parents reported that they felt alone and isolated following the baby's birth and found it difficult to face family and friends. Seven couples reported that they relied heavily on one another and drew closer together. However, in other instances the crisis of the birth separated parents, particularly those who blamed each other for the problem.

These two studies suggest that the emotional reaction of parents to the birth of a less than perfect baby is similar, as Solnit and Stark (1961) suggested, to parental reaction to the death of a child. Shock, denial, anger, and adaptation are stages of the grief process that seemed to be evident in these interviews with parents. A very dramatic difference exists, of course, between the work of mourning the death of a child and the work of mourning the loss of a wished for, perfect baby. The difference is that the work of parents of handicapped babies must continue; continued adaptation to the special needs of the child and acceptance of special responsibilities in caring for the child may be lifelong. The grief process, therefore, is not always neatly time limited. Whereas Kennedy (1970) suggested that an uncomplicated grief and mourning process for parents of babies with birth defects may take as little as six weeks, Drotar et al. (1975) found several families for whom the adaptation process was not complete even after several years. The continuation of the child's life and the demands for care make the death-of-a-child analogy less than perfect. It is encouraging to note the success with which several parents in these studies adapted to their children's special needs and responsibilities. Many mothers emphasized the baby's normalcy and strengths and expressed satisfaction with their ability to care for the child.

## EARLY PARENTING RESPONSES

In addition to exploring the feelings of parents, some studies have observed the behaviors of parents with handicapped infants during the first days and weeks of the baby's life. Researchers have hypothesized that the mother-child interaction may be atypical not only because of grief reactions of the mother but also because of (1) the infant's inability to "take in," to thrive, and to feel comfort and (2) the mother's difficulty in providing maternal care because of the special needs of the baby (Gudermuth, 1975).

A dramatic example of how a handicapping condition in an infant can disturb the mother-child relationship was reported by Freedman, Fox-Kalenda, and Brown (1970). These researchers reviewed the first 18 months of life of a baby multihandicapped because of maternal rubella. The typical posture of the baby was an arched back with the head retracted; he was therefore difficult to carry and to cuddle. He was ill much of the time and was difficult to feed as well as to handle. Because of feeding problems, the mother had to feed him round the clock every three hours for several months. At 18 months he still had to be held in his mother's lap to be fed solids. Although this mother spent a great deal of time with the child, it was clear to the observers that the child care was carried out in a perfunctory manner. When the child failed to respond to her caregiving or opposed her approaches with irritation, she was quickly discouraged. She did much for him but little with him and described the baby as a child who "doesn't like to be bothered."

Similar examples of poor quality mother-child interaction caused by the infant's inability to respond in typical ways and by the unusual demands on the mother for child care can be found in other studies. Gudermuth (1975) investigated the early experiences of mothers with infants with congenital heart disease. In this study, eight mothers of young children attending a cardiology clinic of an urban children's hospital were interviewed regarding their infants' feeding behavior and activity patterns. There was a discrepancy noted between mothers' comments that everything was fine and clinical findings. For example, as a group the mothers described their children as good eaters, yet two children were below the third percentile in weight for their age and sex and an additional four children were below the tenth percentile. Gudermuth concluded that questions about an infant's thriving are threatening because they seem to be related to maternal competence. In spite of the rating of "no problems," the mothers interviewed in this study expressed a strong wish for more concrete information about daily care of the handicapped infants and expressed gratitude for the specific advice that was given in the hospital.

The initial behavioral responses of five mothers toward their infants with birth defects were examined by Mercer (1974). The infants in this study had the following problems at birth: Apert's syndrome, a third naris, Down's syndrome, absence of fingers, and cleft lip. The mothers were interviewed in the hospital at the infant's feeding time during the first eight days of the baby's life, weekly for the first month, and at home at two months and at three months. The investigator recorded verbal and nonverbal responses toward the baby, including general body movements and interactional behaviors. The data were then analyzed by action-interaction units and were classified as maternal assessment, maternal contact, and maternal care activities.

Maternal assessments were the mother's expressed perceptions and appraisals of the infant's appearance or function. Maternal contact behaviors included communicative responses to the infant with the face, hands, or body. Maternal care activities included mothering acts connoting responsiveness or unresponsiveness to baby's cues in acts such as feeding or burping and the seeking of information about the child's condition or care. Interrater reliability scores on a sample of protocols for action-interaction units and categorizations ranged from .73 to .82.

According to Mercer (1974), assessment behaviors increased after the first eight days and remained constant. Examples of assessment behavior included remarks such as the following: "I'm glad her mouth is small"; "Her hands look like claws" (p. 135). Percentage of total contact behaviors indicated that aversion contact behaviors were higher at three months than during the first week. This finding suggests that mothers feel unreadiness and ambivalence about total involvement with the infant. The attachment (bonding) process between the mother and child did not show an increase during the first three months of the infant's life. This finding is consistent with the Drotar et al. (1975) suggestion that the attachment process can be a lengthy one for some parents of handicapped infants.

## VARIABLES AFFECTING PARENTAL REACTION TO THE BIRTH OF A HANDICAPPED CHILD

Studies that have examined theories of grief and mourning at the birth of a handicapped child and early parenting responses have provided a heightened understanding of how parents react to this crisis. Although the theory of how parents as a group respond is helpful, it is of critical importance that clinicians consider individual differences and be sensitive to individual needs at this difficult time. Parks (1977) suggested that the clinician assess the parents' ability to handle the crisis situation by looking at several variables. What strengths do the parents have? Do they have any particular limitations? What social and family supports are available to them? Are there immediate concerns other than the birth of the handicapped child? This section of the chapter will review research that explored two variables that may influence the individual parent's reaction. These variables are the sex of the parent and the type and severity of the birth defect.

## Mothers and Fathers

Several studies purporting to focus on the parents of children with defects predominantly described the reactions of mothers (i.e., Kennedy, 1970), with only a few accounts by mothers of fathers' reactions (i.e., Johns, 1971). A few studies have attempted to look at the reactions of fathers and at differences between mothers and fathers in their reaction to the birth of a handicapped baby.

Mercer (1974) provided two case studies of fathers' early responses to the birth of a daughter with a defect. The early behaviors of the two fathers of comparable age, social class, and professional education reflected two different reaction patterns. The father of a baby with a cleft lip did not express grief openly nor could he permit his wife's expression of grief. The wife felt she had had to support and help the father at this time. The father seemed to have a need to affirm his masculinity by such behaviors as announcing that he "deposited the sperm" that made the baby and asking the interviewer whether he had sex appeal. The second father, whose baby daughter was born with Down's syndrome, was able to express grief but also to look beyond his own grief to express empathy toward his wife and to inquire about his baby's needs. These two fathers, who were similar in many ways, exhibited two different patterns of adaptation to a crisis situation. The father who perceived expressions of grief as unacceptable and whose identity was threatened by the birth of a daughter with a defect was unable to be empathetic or supportive of others. The father who perceived expressions of grief as acceptable and whose identity was not threatened approached the situation more realistically. Past psychosocial experiences may be the important variables in determining the response to this crisis situation.

Differences between the reactions of mothers and fathers have been explored, and the results have been inconsistent. Two British studies examined parental reactions to the birth of babies with spina bifida. Walker, Thomas, and Russell (1971) found little difference between mothers and fathers. Both the mothers and fathers were found to suffer grief, confusion, and physical exhaustion during the first days and weeks following the birth of the spina bifida baby. In another study, however, fathers appeared to be more distressed than mothers by the news that the baby had a defect. It was later learned, however, that the mothers had not absorbed the reality of the event during the first three days (Hare et al., 1966). In an American study, Ehlers (1966) found that mothers reported feelings of shock, disbelief, and grief at the diagnosis of mental retardation whereas fathers were described as expressing anger at the diagnosis, insisting that nothing could be wrong with the child.

A questionnaire was developed by Gumz and Gubrium (1972) to elicit information about the attitudes, perceptions, and beliefs of mothers and fathers of mentally retarded children. Particular emphasis was placed on parents' attitudes toward the crisis of having a handicapped child and on what future roles they foresaw for themselves in the care of the child. There was a tendency for fathers to perceive the child in terms of specific goals—helping the child develop independence, find appropriate job opportunities, etc. The mothers were more likely to think of their roles in interpersonal terms; they saw themselves as managing tensions among different family members. In general, the mothers exhibited more emotional reactions to hearing the diagnosis of mental retardation. This was attributed to mothers' having a clearer anticipation of the time involved in caring for the child, the emotional strain, and problems in maintaining family harmony and integration. In summary, studies that compared reactions of mothers and fathers to the crisis of the birth of a handicapped child have suggested that mothers and fathers may respond differently, but it is not yet clear what those differences are.

## Type and Severity of Birth Defect

Although there may be similarities in the reactions of parents to the birth of a handicapped baby regardless of the type or severity of the handicap, it would seem that the nature of the handicap itself would have some bearing on the parental reaction. Easson (1966) suggested that negative parental reaction may be greatest for defects that affect facial or genital appearance. This clinician presented case studies that suggested that children with congenital facial defects faced profound family and emotional reactions that compounded their physical difficulties. Genital anomalies create uncertainty about anatomical and physiological sex, with resultant impairment of sexual identity and self-concept development.

Other factors that might influence the emotional reaction to the defect include the correctability of the defect, its visibility, and its effect on speech, intellectual functioning, and activities of daily living. In an attempt to understand how handicapping conditions are perceived by parents, Barsch (1964) asked 189 mothers and 122 fathers of handicapped children to rank 10 handicapping conditions in order of severity. There was a marked concordance among the parents in ranking cerebral palsy, mental retardation, mental illness, and brain injury as the most severe problems that could be experienced by a child. The other conditions, in order of rated severity, were blindness, epilepsy, deafness, polio, heart disease, and diabetes. The conditions with the most severe rankings do impair intellectual functioning and activities of daily living, are lifelong in nature, and are more visible than heart disease and diabetes, the conditions rated as least severe. A comparison of rankings by parents of nonhandicapped children showed essentially the same order of severity.

An interaction between social class and severity of handicap has been noted by Grossman (1972). In this intensive study of 83 families with a mentally or physically handicapped child, Grossman found that for upper-class men, the more serious the physical handicap, the better their acceptance of the child. The upper-class family with a physically handicapped child seems to have less confusion about its caregiving role than the upper-class family with a less obviously handicapped child. For lower-class families who do not have the financial resources to provide for the physical demands of a severely handicapped child comfortably, the presence of a physical handicap makes adjustment more difficult for the family.

## COMMUNICATING THE DIAGNOSIS

As has been noted, numerous difficulties and challenges face the parents of babies born with handicaps. The first hurdle that must be faced by parents is the acceptance and understanding of the diagnosis of a handicapping condition. This section will review studies that have explored how parents were told that there was something wrong with their baby, their satisfaction with how this difficult information was presented, and how they wish they had been told.

### How Parents Are Told

Interviews with parents shortly after the time of diagnosis, retrospective interviews, and retrospective questionnaires have been the typical ways of gathering information about how initial information about a baby's handicapping condition was presented. In a British study, Johns (1971) conducted three formal interviews each of one hour's duration with 12 mothers of babies with congenital anomalies. The first interview took place in the hospital immediately after the mother was informed of the problem; this was typically within 24 hours of delivery. The second interview was held at the hospital during a return visit at three months; the final interview took place at home at six months. The kinds of congenital abnormalities represented in this group of babies included club foot, congenital heart disease, cleft palate, hydrocephalus, and Down's syndrome. These 12 babies represented the total sample of babies with a congenital abnormality born within a three-month period in a city hospital in Great Britain. No mother recalled any reference to the child's abnormality at the time of delivery. Four were informed by their husbands and reported that they were glad to have had the news in this manner. The other eight mothers were told of the baby's difficulty while they were on the maternity ward by a hospital staff member, typically not a physician and typically not a person known by the mother. The mothers in this group expressed embarrassment at the lack of privacy in receiving this news and dissatisfaction with the length of time they had to wait to talk to the physician about the problem. There was a unanimous expression of need for a detailed discussion with the doctor regarding the baby's problem even though no mother reported directly requesting such a conference.

In contrast to this British study in which physicians were absent and longed for, studies in the United States identified the physician almost universally as the bearer of this difficult news. In a survey of 414 parents of children with Down's syndrome, 76% reported that a physician first notified the parent of the diagnosis (Pueschel & Murphy, 1976). It is of note that in many cases the diagnosis was communicated to the mother only; 35% of the fathers reported that they were informed of the baby's problems by their spouse. Nurses, social workers, medical students, interns, consultants, and relatives were occasionally mentioned as those who gave the information. Members of the National Association of Retarded Citizens were invited to correspond with Zwerling (1954) regarding the circumstances of their first learning of the diagnosis of mental retardation in their child. Many respondents (33 of 85) referred to the importance of the attitude of the physician: "The points I remember were his gentle treatment of us, his choice of words so as to avoid the obnoxious ones" (p. 471).

The importance of the attitude of the physician is dramatically emphasized in examples of extreme insensitivity. One parent reported that her doctor had commented about her Down's syndrome daughter that "they make nice pets around the house" (p. 471). Another physician reported the diagnosis of Down's with tears running down his cheeks, wringing his hands, and saying, "Something is terribly, terribly wrong" (p. 471).

The time when the mother and father are told of the handicapping condition has also been studied. In reviewing parents' reactions to the birth of children with cleft palate, Tisza and Gumpertz (1962) reported case studies in which information was delayed following delivery. One mother was reported to have waited for three days to see her baby without being told what was wrong. Another, whose baby was sent to another hospital for surgery before she was informed, imagined far worse handicaps than the actual cleft lip and palate. This kind of delay of information is not the norm. In a review of counseling practices with parents of babies with Down's syndrome, Pueschel and Murphy (1976) found that 28% of parents were informed of the diagnosis within the first day of the baby's life; an additional 27% were informed within the first week. In one-third of the cases, however, the diagnosis was communicated to the parents after the child was older than 30 days. Nearly one-half of the parents of Down's syndrome babies reported that professionals had presented the diagnosis in a sympathetic manner; 25% of parents said that the physician was abrupt and blunt. Some parents commented that they were given very little information and that the physician was evasive; two parents were told of their child's condition by mail.

In recent years, physicians seem to be doing a more comprehensive job in communicating the nature and causes of congenital handicaps. In contrast to Thurston's (1963) finding that only 4% of his sample understood the nature and cause of their child's disability or Zwerling's (1954) and Tisza and Gumpertz's (1962) examples of extreme insensitivity, a 1976 survey by Abramson, Gravink, Abramson, and Sommers (1977) found that 18% of the sample of 215 families felt that they had received informative and sympathetic advice and an additional 27% felt that advice to be objective and accurate.

## Parental Satisfaction with the Communication of the Diagnosis

Parental dissatisfaction with the way they were informed has been confirmed by several studies. Zwerling (1954) noted that parents viewed hasty and casual diagnosis with bitterness. Fifty-one percent of the 215 families with a mentally retarded child surveyed by Abramson et al. (1977) reported that they were very dissatisfied with or uncertain about the advice they had received. Tizard and Grad (1964) reported that 14% of the cases in their sample had been poorly handled, 41% had some unsatisfactory features, and 45% were satisfactorily handled.

Price-Bonham and Addison's (1978) review pointed to several major errors in informing parents of birth defects:

1. Delay in defining the problem
2. False encouragement of parents
3. Too much advice on matters such as institutionalization (Jensen, 1960)
4. Abruptness
5. Being hurried
6. Lack of interest
7. Hesitancy to communicate (Koch et al., 1959)

Some researchers and theorists have attributed parental dissatisfaction with how information was presented to hostility toward the bearer of bad news. Baum (1962) described some parents who "make unreasonable demands, are irritable, and ungrateful to those who try to respond" (p. 357). Solnit and Stark (1961) interpreted these parental reactions as a stage in the process of mourning. Zuk (1960) described parental hostility toward the physician as a displaced reaction to frustration at the existence of the handicapped child.

Some theorists and researchers have noted, however, that there may be a reality base to parental hostility: professionals are sometimes harsh and insensitive. Waechter (1970) postulated that nurses and other health care professionals may be abrupt or seemingly insensitive because of feelings of inadequacy and helplessness in the face of irreversible handicaps. Some physicians may be seemingly insensitive because of limited training and exposure in this area (Olshansky, Johnson, & Sternfeld, 1964).

The data suggest that attempting to remain the objective scientist, minimize symptoms, or give too much advice too soon about institutionalization may be the physician's defense against getting caught up in problems that are painful and that have no easy solutions. In contrast, when a contact is established with one of the early intervention programs that are now available to handicapped children and their families, parental responses are enthusiastic (Abramson et al., 1977). It would seem that the positive action offered by an early intervention program offers a ray of hope after the initially distressing diagnosis.

## How Parents Would Like to Be Told

Parents would like to be told about their baby's birth defect as early as possible. Parents of mentally retarded children who wrote to Zwerling (1954) were in agreement that parents should be told as soon as a problem is suspected. Great anger was expressed about professionals' attempts to minimize symptoms or to suggest that the child would catch up or grow out of a handicap. Many parents in the Pueschel and Murphy (1976) study of Down's syndrome families commented that they would have preferred to be told of their child's condition soon after birth. The most resentful parents are those who have not been told early; the most appreciative parents are those who have been told soon after the child's birth (Drillien & Wolkinson, 1964).

There is no consensus among parents as to whether parents should be told together or separately. Tizard and Grad (1964) found that 97% of 128 mothers believed that the mother should be told as soon as possible and then she should tell her husband. The mothers in the Johns (1971) study were grateful that they had been told by their spouses. Many parents in the Pueschel & Murphy (1976) study stressed the fact that both parents should be present during the initial discussion with the physician as they could offer support to one another. In this group, both parents were told together of the child's condition in only 20% of the cases; in most instances the diagnosis was made while only one parent was present. Some physicians talked to the mother since she was available in the hospital when they made rounds. Other professionals assumed the father to be the "stronger" of the two parents and found it easier to tell him first.

*Parents would like complete, practical information about the handicapping condition.* The mothers interviewed by Johns (1971) generated a list of questions for which they wished they had answers. How common is this condition? Do external abnormalities mean that there are things wrong inside the baby? Should I fear another pregnancy? What procedures or treatments are available to help with this condition? Zwerling's (1954) parents reported the need for continuing positive advice of a practical nature on the day-to-day handling of problems. For conditions for which corrective procedures and rehabilitative measures exist, guidance about what to expect, timetables, and resources is needed (Tisza & Gumpertz, 1962).

*What is not needed is premature urging to institutionalize the baby.* Parents in Zwerling's (1954) study commented that institutionalization was presented to them as a way to "put away" a child rather than as a positive procedure for the child's management and care. This kind of professional pressure has been more common in previous years (Jensen, 1960). Recent studies (such as Pueschel & Murphy, 1976) have found that only a few physicians push for immediate institutionalization of a handicapped baby. The trends of better community services, nonavailability of institutional care, and increased understanding of the valued role a handicapped child can play in a family have made this kind of early recommendation inappropriate.

## EVALUATION OF THE RESEARCH

The research that has been reviewed here has been drawn from several disciplines: medicine, nursing, psychology, social work, and special education. This interdisciplinary focus suggests that the topic is one of concern for a number of professionals, yet the research is characterized by a number of methodological problems. Among these problems are the lack of control groups, possible sampling errors, other uncontrolled variables, and questionable methods of collecting data.

Only one study reviewed here used a control group. Barsch's (1964) study of the ranking of severity of handicaps by parents compared ratings by parents of handicapped children with ratings by parents of nonhandicapped children. The other studies focused exclusively on the reactions of parents whose babies who were handicapped. These studies found that the time period following the birth of a less than perfect baby is stressful for parents. Since other research has indicated that the postpartum period may be difficult for many parents (see Chapter 4), the unique aspects of the crisis for parents of handicapped babies cannot be unequivocally established until parental reactions are compared to those of parents of non-handicapped babies. Of special interest would be comparisons with parents of premature infants and with parents of newborns of undesired gender (e.g., "We wanted a girl, but he's a boy").

The low incidence of birth defects in general and of specific congenital anomalies in particular makes research with large groups of subjects quite difficult. Several studies reported the reactions of very small groups: Mercer (1974) focused on 5 mothers and 2 fathers; Johns (1971) worked with 12 mothers; Gudermuth (1975) worked with 8 mothers. It may be difficult to draw valid conclusions about behavior from such small groups. In addition to their small size, the groups often include different types of birth defects (Drotar et al., 1975; Kennedy, 1970). Since it has been suggested that parental reaction may be influenced by the visibility, location, permanence, and severity of the defect, researchers should probably control for this variable as did Gudermuth (1975) and Pueschel and Murphy (1976). Since it has been noted also that mothers and fathers may differ in their responses (Ehlers, 1966; Gumz & Gubrium, 1972), the sex of the parent should also be considered. Some studies have drawn from a special segment of the population of parents of handicapped babies: Zwerling's (1954) parents belonged to the National Association for Retarded Citizens, for example. The reactions of parents in special groups or parents whose children are involved in special treatment programs may not be generalizable to parents who have not chosen to use such services or who have not had the opportunity to do so.

Methods for collecting data have relied heavily on interviewing techniques, sometimes described as semistructured (Kennedy, 1970). Problems with this method include the possibility that questioning may lead the respondent to answer in such a way as to fit a preconceived model. In addition, some interviews are retrospective in nature; Droter et al. (1975) interviewed some parents within the first week of life of the handicapped baby but did not interview others until several years after the birth. Retrospective data are difficult to interpret in that parents may have difficulty remembering events and feelings, and the accuracy of the memories is difficult to verify.

It is easier to criticize the available research than it is to suggest research strategies that are closer to the ideal. The vulnerability of parents of newborns with birth defects makes the sensitive researcher reluctant to intrude with elaborate questionnaires or to set up well-controlled clinical studies. The best research about parental responses to the birth of a handicapped child will continue to be sensitive to the needs of the parents. Better research might include longitudinal work with small numbers of families to observe their changes in response over time, videotaping parent-child interactions as a routine part of the hospital stay and early care of all newborns, greater attention to interrater reliability, and comparisons of different support strategies for families with handicapped babies.

## RECOMMENDATIONS FOR PROFESSIONALS CARING FOR PARENTS OF HANDICAPPED BABIES

There is little joy in communicating to parents the news that a longed for baby is imperfect and that the problems may be serious and lifelong in nature. There may be satisfaction, however, in helping those parents muster available resources to deal with this difficult crisis and help the handicapped infant become the best he or she can be. The following recommendations are offered to those who provide the initial diagnosis and to those who give continuing support to families with less than perfect babies:

1. The initial diagnosis should be communicated by a physician who has an established relationship with the parent(s). If the pediatrician is new to the family, it would be good for the obstetrician to be involved in the initial conference.
2. Information about a handicapping condition should be shared with the parent(s) at the earliest possible time and an opportunity for parents to ask questions should be provided.
3. As there is no consensus among parents or professionals as to which parent should be told first, it is recommended that this decision be made on an individual basis by someone who knows the family well.
4. It is advisable initially to have one brief meeting to share the diagnosis and its most important implications and at that time set up a second meeting time (for the next day or within the week) to discuss in detail the nature, cause (if known), and prognosis of the condition with both parents.
5. It is essential that information be presented in a tactful, sympathetic, and accurate manner. Evasions and attempts to minimize symptoms are not appreciated by parents. Real understanding for the grief and stress that parents are undergoing must be expressed. Kanner (1953) stated that what parents need most is "sympathetic endorsement of themselves, of their human and parental competence, of their right not to blame themselves for what has happened" (p. 375).
6. An early description of available medical or surgical treatment for correctable problems is needed. Included here should be information about what kind of treatment is available, what the likely outcome will be, the timetable for treatment, and the steps the parents must take to arrange for such treatment.
7. Positive assistance should be offered to families of even the most severely disabled child. Knowledge of local early intervention programs should be shared; the names of contact persons should be given. If special

instruction is needed for the daily care of the infant (for example, feeding techniques for cleft palate babies), this instruction should be provided in the hospital.

8. Genetic counseling should be made available to the family if they request it or if the nature of the baby's handicapping condition suggests that such counseling is advisable.

9. An offer should be made by the professional to share information about the baby's condition with siblings, grandparents, or other significant family members.

10. Ongoing support to the family from members of the hospital staff (psychologist, social worker, nurse), early intervention programs, and other appropriate resources should be offered.

11. Contact with other families who have dealt with similar difficulties in constructive ways is often helpful (Flint & Deloach, 1975).

12. Professionals must keep in close touch with available resources in the community and must keep abreast of current trends in community acceptance of handicapped persons. In recent years, increased sensitivity to the special needs of handicapped persons and their families and increased community resources for education and training make the chances of the handicapped child's becoming the best he or she can be considerably brighter.

13. Much of what we are suggesting here relates to the conveying of accurate information to the parents. The importance of such information and the potential utility of it have been suggested as a significant component of many types of psychological intervention and counseling (Selby & Calhoun, in press). Another form of information that professionals may find useful to convey involves the types of emotional reactions parents are likely to experience. The research and theory summarized in this chapter should provide a useful departure point for discussing the sorts of psychological responses parents are likely to experience. We think it imperative, however, that as part of the responsibility of conveying accurate information in a sensitive manner, the professional who works with parents of handicapped children be highly knowledgeable about the medical aspects of the child's handicap and maintain a complete and current knowledge of research on the psychological reactions of parents to the birth of a handicapped baby.

## REFERENCES

ABRAMSON, P. R., GRAVINK, M. J., ABRAMSON, L. M., and SOMMERS, D. Early diagnosis and intervention of retardation: a survey of parental reactions concerning the quality of services rendered. *Mental Retardation,* 1977, *15,* 28–31.

APGAR, V., and BECK, J. *Is my baby all right?* New York: Pocket Books, 1974.

BARSCH, R. H. The handicapped scale among parents of handicapped children. *American Journal of Public Health,* 1964, *54,* 1560–1567.

Baum, M. H. Some dynamic factors affecting family adjustment to the handicapped child. *Exceptional Children,* 1962, *28,* 387–392.

Drillien, C. M., and Wolkinson, E. M. Mongolism: when should parents be told? *British Medical Journal,* 1964, *2,* 1306.

Drotar, D., Baskiewicz, A., Irvin, N., Kennell, J., and Klaus, M. The adaptation of parents to the birth of an infant with a congenital malformation: a hypothetical model. *Pediatrics,* 1975, *56,* 710–717.

Easson, W. M. Psychopathological environmental reaction to congenital defect. *Journal of Nervous and Mental Disease.* 1966, *142,* 453–459.

Ehlers, W. H. *Mothers of retarded children: how they feel, where they find help.* Springfield: Charles C Thomas, 1966.

Flint, W., and DeLoach, C. A parent involvement program model for handicapped children and their parents. *Exceptional Children,* 1975, *41,* 556–557.

Freedman, D. A., Fox-Kalenda, B. J., and Brown, S. L. A multihandicapped rubella baby: the first 18 months. *Journal of the American Academy of Child Psychiatry,* 1970, *9,* 298–317.

Grossman, F. K. *Brothers and sisters of retarded children.* Syracuse: Syracuse University Press, 1972.

Gudermuth, S. Mothers' reports of early experiences of infants with congenital heart disease. *Maternal-Child Nursing Journal,* 1975, *4,* 155–164.

Gumz, E. J., and Gubrium, J. Comparative parental perceptions of a mentally retarded child. *American Journal of Mental Deficiency,* 1972, *77,* 175–177.

Hare, E. H., Lawrence, K. M., Payne, H., and Rawnsley, K. Spina bifida cystica and family stress. *British Medical Journal,* 1966, *2,* 757.

Jensen, R. A. The clinical management of the mentally retarded child and his parents. *American Journal of Mental Deficiency,* 1960, *66,* 830–833.

Johns, N. Family reactions to the birth of a child with a congenital abnormality. *Medical Journal of Australia,* 1971, *1,* 277–282.

Kanner, L. Parents' feeling about retarded children. *American Journal of Mental Deficiency,* 1953, *57,* 375–383.

Kennedy, J. F. Maternal reactions to the birth of a defective baby. *Social Casework,* 1970, *51,* 410–416.

Koch, R., Grailiker, B. V., Sands, R., and Parmelee, A. H. Attitude survey of parents with mentally retarded children: evaluation of parental satisfaction with medical care of a retarded child. *Pediatrics,* 1959, *23,* 582–584.

Meadow, K. P., and Meadow, R. Changing role perceptions for parents of handicapped children. *Exceptional Children,* 1971, *38,* 21–27.

Mercer, R. T. Mothers' responses to their infants with defects. *Nursing Research,* 1974, *23,* 133–137.

———. Two fathers' early responses to the birth of a daughter with a defect. *Maternal-Child Nursing Journal,* 1974, *3,* 77–86.

Olshansky, S., Johnson, G. C., and Sternfeld, L. Attitudes of some GP's toward institutionalizing mentally retarded children. In *Institutionalizing mentally retarded children: attitudes of some physicians.* Washington, D.C.: U.S. Government Printing Office, 1964.

Parks, R. M. Parental reactions to the birth of a handicapped child. *Health and Social Work,* 1977, *2,* 51–66.

Price-Bonham, S., and Addison, S. Families and mentally retarded children: emphasis on the father. *Family Coordinator,* 1978, *27,* 221–230.

Pueschel, S. M., and Murphy, A. Assessment of counseling practices at the birth of a child with Down's Syndrome. *American Journal of Mental Deficiency,* 1976, *81,* 325–330.

Selby, J. W., and Calhoun, L. G. The psychodidactic element of psychological intervention: an undervalued and underdeveloped treatment tool. *Professional Psychology,* in press.

SOLNIT, A. J., and STARK, M. H. Mourning and the birth of a defective child. *Psychoanalytic Study of the Child,* 1961, *16,* 523–537.

THURSTON, J. R. Counseling the parents of mentally retarded children. *Training School Bulletin,* 1963, *60,* 113–117.

TISZA, V. B., and GUMPERTZ, E. The parents' reaction to the birth and early care of children with cleft palate. *Pediatrics,* 1962, *30,* 86–90.

TIZARD, J., and GRAD, J. *The mentally handicapped and their families: a social survey.* New York: Oxford University Press, 1964.

WAECHTER, E. H. The birth of an exceptional child. *Nursing Forum,* 1970, *9,* 202–216.

WALKER, J. H., THOMAS, M., and RUSSELL, I. T. Spina bifida—and the parents. *Developmental Medicine and Child Neurology,* 1971, *13,* 466.

ZUK, G. H. The influence of anger and guilt on parents of handicapped children. Paper presented to the United Cerebral Palsy Association, Chicago, 1960.

ZWERLING, I. Initial counseling of parents with mentally retarded children. *Journal of Pediatrics,* 1954, *44,* 469–479.

# Chapter 7

# Psychological Implications of Early Parent–Neonate Interactions

THE NEWBORN HAS BEEN THE FOCUS of a dramatically increasing amount of theoretical speculation and research by various professional groups. The rapid changes in the neonate's motor and sensory capabilities have been studied for decades; however, until recently, little attention has been focused on the social world of the neonate. The development of improved neonatal assessment procedures such as the Brazelton Neonatal Assessment Scale (Brazelton, 1973) has overcome many of the methodological obstacles to a more accurate and complete understanding of the newborn's role in the parent-infant interaction (St. Clair, 1978). The present chapter reviews the available data on early social interaction of neonates. Particular emphasis is given to parent-infant interactions during the immediate postpartum period.

Historically, infants have often been viewed as receptive and passive parts of parent-child interactions. Theorists developed and relied upon a unidirectional model of social influence, with the parent's behavior, particularly that of the mother, affecting the infant, and the infant's behavior having little of significant impact on the parent. Parents and professionals readily assumed that since the human newborn is small, inexperienced, and apparently possesses only the crudest of social skills, it is the parents who exert virtually total control over the course of their social interactions with their offspring. Yet, Rheingold (1966), among others, noted that "the amount of attention and the number of responses directed to the infant are enormous—out of all proportion to his age, size and accomplishments" (p. 12). She proposed a truly interactive model of early social interaction in which the effect of the infant on the behavior of both parents is recognized. Specifically, Rheingold asserted that four principles of infant behavior have emerged from research and that these principles must be acknowledged in order truly to understand the development of social behavior in infants. First, the human infant, from the earliest moments of life, is able to respond to a wide variety of social and nonsocial stimuli. Second, the human infant is from birth an active rather than a passive creature. Third, the infant can and will change his or her behavior in response to environmental demands. Fourth, the human infant can and will modify the behavior of others interacting with him or her. Other researchers have concurred with the validity and significance of these principles (e.g., Bell, 1968, 1971, 1974; Klaus & Kennell, 1976, 1977). Thus, the simple unidirectional model of early interaction, which does not recognize that the control of the social world of the newborn is shared by parent and infant, may be not only incomplete but also inaccurate.

A number of theoretical and practical issues have arisen as a consequence of the altered perspective on early parent-infant interaction. To understand these issues, it is necessary to document the impact of prenatal and postdelivery factors on the interaction of neonate and parents following parturition and to clarify the nature of the reciprocal social interactions during the early postpartum period. In the present chapter, these matters will be discussed in some detail.

## FACTORS AFFECTING EARLY SOCIAL INTERACTION

### Infant Characteristics

Several infant characteristics, some present prior to birth, have been found to significantly influence the course of parent-infant interactions after delivery. At birth, human infants differ in both appearance and action. These differences can be attributed to genetic factors (which especially determine much of the physical appearance of the infant), constitutional factors (which especially influence the behavior of the infant), and environmental intrusions experienced by the infant in utero (which may influence appearance and/or behavior after birth).

Whether a particular infant characteristic is the product solely of heredity, physical structure and function, or environmental intrusion is often impossible to determine. Nevertheless, researchers have found that on specific behavioral dimensions not attributable to learning human infants usually differ. Bell (1968) noted that human newborns differ from one another on the behavioral dimensions of activity level (or assertiveness) and degree of social orientation (responsiveness to others). Furthermore, the neonate's relative levels of activity and social orientation appear remarkably stable over time. Other researchers have noted similar behavioral dimensions that distinguish human infants and remain stable over time (e.g. Scarr, 1966, 1969). The infant's relative levels of assertiveness and social orientation are independent of each other such that the level of one does not predict the level of the other. In addition, these differences can be identified almost as soon as the effect of the birth trauma and obstetrical medication has subsided. This finding has led researchers to conclude that the different levels of assertiveness and social orientation cannot be readily ascribed to learning but rather to factors operating before delivery. For example, Walters (1965) found that the amount of fetal activity reported by mothers during the last trimester of pregnancy was predictive of their infants' motor development scores on the Gesell Development Schedules at 12, 24, and 36 weeks. This finding is consistent with the hypothesis of stable, unlearned differences in motor activity in human infants.

Although learning appears to have little to do with determining the infant's initial levels of assertiveness and social orientation, postdelivery experience seems to contribute strongly to the maintenance of these behavioral differences among infants. The manner in which parents and other adults react to the newborn is determined in part by how that newborn is behaving. The neonate with a low level of assertiveness will elicit caretaking styles from adults different from those commanded by a neonate high in assertiveness. The neonate high in social orientation, being more of a "cuddler," will be treated differently from the low social orientation neonate. In this way, the unlearned behavior of the neonate affects postdelivery social experiences.

The parent responds not only to how the infant behaves but also to the gender and appearance of the infant. Male and female infants elicit somewhat different parenting responses. These differences may reflect behavioral differences between male and female newborns, along with culturally determined expectations regarding the differential treatment of sons and daughters.

Bell and Costello (1964), in a pioneering study of unlearned sex differences in behavior, tested neonates on several measures of tactile sensitivity. Female newborns were found to be more reactive to the removal of a cover blanket and to the stimulation of the abdomen with an air jet. This demonstration of lower thresholds of touch in female neonates implied that female neonates need less tactile stimulation from parents to elicit the same response that high stimulation elicits from male neonates. Thus, the higher activity levels of male neonates reconfirmed in recent research (Phillips, King, & Dubois, 1978), and the rougher, more active interactions between parents and sons may be the result in part of differential levels of infant sensitivity that are detectible before sex role training has begun (Weller &

Bell, 1965). Consistent with this hypothesis, Brown, Bakeman, Snyder, Fredrickson, Morgan and Helper (1975) found that male newborns were rubbed, patted, touched, kissed, rocked and talked to by their mothers more frequently than were female newborns, and Parke, O'Leary and West (1972) report that both parents touched male neonates more than female neonates. Male newborns appeared to elicit more stimulation in part because they were generally more irritable and slept less than female newborns (Moss 1969). However, as Osofsky and O'Connell (1977) have recently noted, the high degree of social responsivity in female infants appears to contribute to the consistent finding of more one-to-one eye contact between female infants and their mothers. It appears that female infants are more responsive to stimulation of distance receptors (i.e., eyes, ears) than are male newborns and that this differential sensitivity to such stimulation may be a major factor in differential treatment of newborn sons and daughters by parents.

Beyond gender, the infant's appearance may influence his or her social interactions. Parke and Sawin (1975) reported that, while the mother's response to her newborn may not be significantly affected by the "cuteness" of the neonate, the father of the cute newborn is more responsive to him or her than is the father of the less than cute newborn. Brown and Bakeman (1977) contended that the unattractiveness of the premature neonate is responsible, in part, for the low maternal involvement often noted with such infants.

In sum, the nature of the post-partum interaction between parent and infant can be significantly influenced by characteristics of the child determined before delivery. The neonate's gender, appearance, and to some extent, his or her social behavior are determined prior to birth.

## Parental Characteristics

The nature of the early interactions between parent and infant is, of course, not exclusively dependent on the characteristics of the infant. A danger of the bidirectional model is the failure to maintain an appreciation of the power of the parent.

Certain parental characteristics may directly influence the offspring's behavior. Parents carry the genetic packages that contribute to the infant's genetic makeup. Maternal drug use, maternal diet during pregnancy, maternal emotional state, age, and parity are related to neonatal behavior.

The sensitivity of the neonate is fragile and the intrusion of drugs during pregnancy and/or at delivery may dramatically impair the infant's response to social stimulation. Although light to moderate amounts of obstetrical medication may not greatly distort the behavior of the newborn (Conway & Brackbill, 1970; Horowitz et al., 1977), there appear to be subtle yet notable effects of such drugs on the neonate (Brazelton, 1969). Tranquilizers, barbiturates, and succinylcholine, a blocking agent, have been found to alter the infant's habituation and orienting responses and his or her cuddliness and smiling throughout the first postpartum month, with the deleterious effects peaking at four weeks (Aleksandrowicz & Aleksandrowicz, 1974). This persistent depression of neonatal responsiveness may then serve to alter parental responsiveness. The groggy mother and depressed infant, unable to respond appropriately to each other during the early hours and days, may be missing the moments most conducive to the establishment of a strong parent-infant bond. We will examine early parent-infant bonding in a later section.

Although legal drugs may influence early social interactions, illegal drug use by the mother may lead to a far more serious disruption of neonatal responsiveness. Newborns of mothers addicted to narcotics have been found to display classic signs of narcotics abstinence, have difficulty orienting toward visual and auditory stimuli, and often fail to be maintained in an alert state—a state quite easily displayed and one that is critical to normal social functioning by neonates born to nonaddicted mothers. These harmful effects to the infant appear to peak at around 48 hours after delivery, with the neonates becoming increasingly irritable and less willing to cuddle (Strauss et al., 1975). Infants of heroin addicts may even die as a consequence of acute withdrawal symptoms. Even when the infant survives, his or her behaviors are not conducive to optimal parent-infant bonding. Reports of the harmful effects on the fetus caused by maternal alcohol consumption (Clarren & Smith, 1978; Little & Streissguth, 1978), tobacco smoking (Garn, Shaw, & McCabe, 1978), and marijuana usage (Staab & Lynch, 1977) have suggested that great care be taken by mothers during pregnancy regarding the type of drug to which they are exposing the unborn child.

Less dramatic parental characteristics also appear to influence postpartum social interaction. Maternal personality characteristics assessed during the newlywed period have been found to predict responsiveness to the infant (Moss, Ryder, & Robson, 1967). Mothers who were in frequent and positive interaction with their own mothers, who accepted the traditional feminine role, and who dwelt on the warm, personal, and rewarding aspects of babies during the newlywed interview were subsequently found to be more responsive to the great and subtle needs of their own infants. On the other hand, mothers who demonstrated a high level of identification with their fathers were found to be less responsive in subsequent interactions with their infants. These factors were found to be especially related to the mother's interaction with her infant within the first few weeks after delivery, with their impact weakening somewhat thereafter. Moss and Robson (1968) further reported that a pregnant woman's statements of interest in her unborn child predict how much mutual face-to-face gazing will subsequently take place between her and her infant during the first month after delivery.

The mother's age appears to be related to her responsiveness to the newborn. In a study involving mothers aged 15–36 years, Wilson (1977) found that older mothers were more responsive to their newborns than were younger mothers. It was suggested that the older women were more emotionally stable and had developed a greater capacity to nurture than characterized the younger women. Wilson also noted that mothers who chose, prior to delivery, to have their infants remain in the hospital room with them as much as possible were more responsive to their newborns than were mothers who did not choose the rooming-in option.

Prior experience with having a baby also appears to influence how the interaction will develop between mother and infant. Firstborn neonates appear to receive more maternal stimulation than do subsequent children (Cohen & Beckwith, 1977; Kilbride, Johnson, & Streissguth, 1977). Furthermore, multiparous mothers have been found to hold stronger beliefs in the power of the newborn to direct mother-infant interaction than did women pregnant for the first time (Lessen-Firestone, 1977). Primiparous mothers planned to direct the course of their interactions with the infant whereas multiparous mothers were more likely to expect the infant to plot the path of the interaction. However, after delivery these first-time mothers became more likely to agree with the multiparas that the newborn is indeed extremely powerful in directing early social interactions.

In sum, parent-infant interaction during the early postpartum period is clearly related to the attitudes and values expressed prior to delivery by the mother (and perhaps even the father). The subsequent interaction is the result of a complex interplay of parental and newborn characteristics, cultural expectations, and, as will be discussed later in this chapter, the timing and setting of the birth.

## POSTPARTUM SOCIAL BEHAVIOR

### The Neonate

The physical, motor, temperamental, and social characteristics of the newborn greatly influence the course of the early interactions between parent and infant. The normal newborn is a remarkably skilled and active person (Appleton, Clifton, & Goldberg, 1975) who possesses sufficient instinctual responses to sustain life. The baby will cry when in pain or when hungry and will suck when provided with food. The infant may hear even before delivery and can localize sound soon after birth. The neonate is usually soothed by low-frequency sounds and by continuous or rhythmic sounds (Birns et al., 1965) and will startle at a sudden noise. The newborn quickly prefers to look at a regular human face rather than at a scrambled face (Lewis, 1969) and usually displays some preference for looking at complex visual stimuli. The newborn can track movement with the eyes and converge them on interesting visual stimuli (Wickelgren, 1967). He or she can also sense the world through touch. Arm movements, sucking, looking, and reflex grasping are all present at birth though not truly coordinated (Ruff & Halton, 1978). Infants can learn exceedingly well as soon as the trauma of delivery (and the effects of any obstetrical medication) has passed. The earliest neonatal period is not only a time of maximum learning efficiency for the infant but also the time of the child's introduction to the entire experience of learning itself.

The newborn also possesses, at or shortly after delivery, skills to achieve active participation in social interaction. The newborn may be drawn by the mother's odor and made alert by her high-pitched voice (Klaus & Kennell, 1976). Neonates may also possess another effective social skill of such subtlety as to elude most caretakers: Condon and Sander (1974) reported that newborns often move their bodies in time with adult speech in an almost imperceptible dance. Such movement may stimulate the adult to continue an interaction or even to escalate it.

In the early postpartum days, the neonate's sensory and motor abilities and instincts are refined and fortified by his or her experience in the social environment. The newborn's remarkable capacity to learn is exemplified in a series of studies that concentrated on the development of early neonatal skills that have social implications.

Although the sucking response has an instinctual basis, Lipsitt, Kaye, and Bosack (1966) found that the newborn learns how to employ and adapt this response to environmental demands in the early days of life. Reinforcement of the sucking response, in the form of dextrose through an artificial nipple, was found significantly to enhance the neonate's rate of sucking on that nipple; the withholding of such reinforcement had the opposite effect. The altered responses displayed by these neonates were gradual, but this study clearly demonstrated that neonates can and do learn to control instinctive behavior quite early in life.

Cohen (1967) found that newborns quickly learned to stop crying at the insertion of the nipple. Nipple pacifiers were inserted into the mouths of crying neonates for three-minute periods. It was found that, with increasing experience with the pacifier, the neonates quieted more quickly at its insertion and cried more quickly when it was removed.

The neonate has been shown to demonstrate similar learning skills in the establishment of other behaviors such as learning to cry to elicit adult attention (Bell & Ainsworth, 1972), learning to show distress by stereotypic mouth and hand movements (Korner, Chuck, & Dontchos, 1968), learning to be soothed and become alert when held to the talking mother's shoulder (Korner & Grobstein, 1966; Thoman, Korner, & Beason-Williams, 1977), and learning to identify the mother and smile to please her (Bower, 1977).

The newborn is able to learn to be controlled and to control his or her environment. Bell (1974) noted that the neonate is not a passive learner and has considerable environmental control in that the newborn defines what it will or will not incorporate by spitting stuff out, turning the head, sleeping when he is supposed to be fed on schedule, showing startle to intense change in stimulation, etc. According to recent, unpublished research by T. G. R. Bower of the University of Edinburgh, the newborn may even be able to imitate some behaviors that he or she is exposed to, thereby stimulating further social interaction.

In an interesting example of the modifying effect of the newborn on parenting behavior, Field (1977) found that mothers infantized their behavior in the presence of newborns. Mothers slowed down, exaggerated, and repeated their own actions; they imitated and highlighted the behaviors of the infant. The mothers and newborns almost conversed, with the infant knowing his or her role (look attentive, sound contented) and the mother quickly learning her role (don't be overactive, be attentive, sound contented).

## The Parents

Parents react in lawful ways to their newborn. The apparent universality of the positive affect and behavior displayed by parents toward their offspring in the period immediately after delivery suggests that some level of instinctual responsiveness may be involved. Harlow (1971) noted that women almost invariably emit "gasps of ecstasy" when shown a picture of an infant rhesus monkey whereas males tend to be unresponsive to the same picture. Harlow contended that "nature not only constructed women to produce babies but has also prepared them from the outset to be mothers" (p. 6).

Other theorists and researchers have suggested that there are indeed species specific responses by fathers and mothers that are displayed during their first interactions with the newborn (e.g., Bowlby, 1958; Klaus & Kennell, 1976). Often at birth women experience a highly positive emotional state and this experience can be contagious for others who witness the birth. These reactions may be especially common among prepared and participating parents (see Chapter 2). The people in the room may display an unreserved, festive elation and show great interest in and attraction toward the infant, especially during the first 15–20 minutes after delivery. The mother often picks up her newborn and, if possible, begins breastfeeding within minutes while others in the room groom her. The ritual does not exclude the father. He can become engrossed in the newborn, experiencing a sense of elation and increased self-esteem. He may engage in a high level of exploration of the newborn when holding the infant. Given the opportunity, fathers perform the same ritualistic routine of fingertip touching of the infant's extremities and massaging of the infant's trunk as does the mother (Newton & Newton, 1962). In fact, the mother's responsiveness to her newborn may be greatly influenced by the father's general responsiveness in the delivery room (Wilson, 1977).

Yet, mothers appear more responsive to the infant than do fathers. Perhaps this is the result of cultural expectations, values, and sex role stereotypes. Others have suggested that the mother's responsiveness is caused at least in part by the presence of specific hormones, related to pregnancy and delivery, that elicit mothering behavior (e.g., Leifer et al., 1972). At present, empirical support for this hypothesis comes from research using animal subjects (e.g., Lott & Rosenblatt, 1969) and the influence of hormones on maternal behavior remains speculative.

## The Sensitive Period

It has been noted that although infants do not typically display a specific affectional bonding tie to another person until after the first half year of life (e.g., Ainsworth, 1973; Schaffer & Emerson, 1964), parental attachment behavior toward the infant may be displayed immediately after delivery. It has been proposed that there exists a sensitive period most conducive to the establishment of strong and lasting parental ties to the newborn. This time of heightened likelihood of attachment appears to be a brief period during and immediately after delivery (Ainsworth, 1973; Hopkins & Vietze, 1977; Klaus & Kennell, 1976; Leifer et al., 1972).

The isolation of newborns from parents in the traditional hospital delivery system has long concerned parents and professionals who contended that parental bonding to the infant may be facilitated by allowing parents to have close contact with their newborn during his or her first hours of life. One observer noted in 1907 that often mothers separated from their newborns quickly lost all interest in them because they were unable to nurse and cherish these infants (Budin 1907). Indeed, infants isolated for a significant amount of time from their mothers immediately after delivery have been found subsequently to be overrepresented in the population of abused children (Parke & Collmer, 1975).

Klaus and Kennell (1976, 1977) have noted that after the trauma of delivery the infant is often in a quiet, alert state that is ideal for eliciting positive social responses from the environment. The neonate will often be in this alert state for the first full hour of life. When the parents are separated from their infant during this period, they are more likely to be initially hesitant and clumsy when allowed interaction with the neonate.

The potency of early interaction was demonstrated in a Swedish study (Greenberg, Rosenberg, & Lind, 1973) in which mothers who were allowed intensive early interaction with their newborns were found to be more confident, feel more competent in caregiving, and appear more sensitive to the crying of the infants than were mothers who were not allowed to have such contact. In a series of American studies by Klaus, Kennell and their colleagues (1976, 1977), it was reported that mothers who were permitted early and extended contact with their infants (i.e., 1 hour of contact within 2 hours after delivery and at least 5 hours of contact on each of the next 3 days) were more playful with the infant, more responsive to him or her, felt more attached to him or her, touched him or her, more, and engaged in more face-to-face interaction with the infant during the first month after delivery than did mothers who experienced normal early contact with their infants (i.e., a glimpse at birth and 20 minutes of contact during each 4-hour period thereafter). When the infants were one year old, the high-contact mothers stayed closer to them and soothed them more than did the normal-contact mothers. When these infants grew to be five-year-old children, those of high-contact mothers had higher IQs and more sophisticated language skills than did the children of the normal-contact mothers (Ringler et al., 1978). Thus, early, extensive mother-neonate interaction was related to remarkable long-term beneficial effects. It may be improper to assume that what occurs in the first hour after delivery directly affects later IQ and language scores. However, it is reasonable to propose that parental interaction styles established during early contacts with the newborn are somewhat resistant to major change and tend to be maintained. It is the style of parenting that is relatively stable over time but traceable to the early interactions that influences the child during at least the first years of life.

In response to the accumulating body of research support for the sensitive period hypothesis, hospital delivery systems have slowly begun to provide mothers with the opportunity for intensive early contact with their infants. In addition, these systems provide the opportunity for fathers and even siblings to interact with the neonate during the sensitive period. In this way, all members of the neonate's immediate family can develop the kinds of interactive skills with regard to the newborn once learned only by the mother. It should be noted, however, that ongoing research projects at the University of Surrey in England by Harry McGurk and at Strathclyde University in Scotland by H. R. Schaffer are finding little support for the importance of the sensitive period.

## An Alternative Delivery Setting

In reaction to a traditional hospital delivery system in which obstetrical medication, institutional sterility, and parental exclusion are often the costs for minimizing delivery and postpartum health risks to mother and infant, Leboyer (1976) proposed an alternative delivery setting. Although it is not yet supported by direct empirical evidence, Leboyer's method appears to maximize the likelihood of positive parent-neonate interaction in the earliest postpartum period. Leboyer argued that neonates born in a traditional system are treated impersonally and display a tragic facial expression and body posture after delivery. He concluded that the body language of the neonate communicates the intense pain and confusion experienced during the first moments after birth.

Leboyer suggested that the delivery setting be "softened." Lights should be lowered, sounds made less discordant, and the tactile stimulation provided to the neonate made less harsh. He stated that when these adjustments are made, the neonate quickly achieves the alert state conducive to positive social interaction (he or she may even smile within moments after delivery) and the parents can more readily respond to the pleasant social signals emitted by their offspring. While still lacking empirical support, Leboyer's "birth without violence" approach to delivery has drawn tentative endorsement from scientific circles.

## The Role of the Father

Although mothers seem especially responsive to the newborn, the father's role during the early postpartum period has been defined as one of relatively detached support. It has been assumed by many that fathers are a biological necessity but a social accident. Nevertheless, men are usually as interested in babies as are women (Feldman & Nash, 1978) and the effect of the newborn on the father has been attracting increasing research interest (Parke & O'Leary, 1976; Parke, O'Leary, & West, 1972; Parke & Sawin, 1975). Researchers are also becoming aware of the power of the newborn to generate so-called second-order effects whereby the newborn may affect relationships among other family members, such as between husband and wife (Clarke-Stewart, 1978; Pedersen, Anderson, & Cain, 1977).

Parke and Sawin (1975) listed four myths regarding the father and his newborn. The first myth is that the father is neither interested in nor involved with the newborn. Second, the father is not as nurturant toward the newborn as is the mother. Third, the father prefers to engage in noncaretaking activities with the newborn and leaves caretaking to the mother. The fourth myth is that the father is not as competent as the mother in caring for the newborn. There has been little empirical support for any of these "rules of fatherhood" and recent research has demonstrated that the father's involvement with the newborn is far more extensive than the 37.7 seconds of verbal interaction per day reported by Rebelsky and Hanks (1971). Since the invention of the baby bottle, the father has the ability to perform any or all of the infant caregiving activities that have been traditionally assigned to the mother.

The series of studies by Parke and his colleagues (Parke & O'Leary, 1976; Parke, O'Leary, & West, 1972; Parke & Sawin, 1975) clearly demonstrated that fathers are usually as involved as mothers with the newborn during the early postpartum period when provided with sufficient opportunity. In fact, fathers were found to hold and rock the newborn more than did mothers when the triad was together. Fathers were also quite nurturant toward the newborn in that they touched, looked at, talked to, and kissed the infant as much as, and in many cases more than, did the mothers. However, fathers were found generally to prefer an actice, awake infant and tended to let the mothers stimulate lethargic and/or drugged infants. Parke also noted the tremendous power of the newborn over the behavior of both parents. If the infant sneezed, coughed, or spit up, both parents oriented quickly toward him or her.

In sum, Parke and O'Leary (1976) stated that "opportunities for early interaction may, in fact, be particularly important for the father who, unlike the mother in the postpartum period, may not be biologically or culturally primed to be responsive to infant cues" (p. 662). Fathers appear to need all the training they can get from their newborn infants.

## LONG-TERM EFFECTS OF EARLY INTERACTION

Early interactions between neonate and parent have been found to be quite predictive of later interaction patterns between child and parent. Blehar, Lieberman, and Ainsworth (1977), for example, reported that early, responsive face-to-face interaction between newborn and mother predicted later infant-mother attachment. It is improbable that such specific events that occur in the early social encounters are direct causes of events that occur years later (Caldwell, 1964). However, early events may contribute to specific perceptions and behaviors that are maintained and perhaps strengthened over time. It is this ongoing pattern of interaction, established early, that results in apparent long-term effects of initial interactive events.

The sensitive period hypothesis, if valid, has clear long-range implications. If neonate and parents interact smoothly during initial encounters, parents may become more strongly attached to their infants and establish positive, effective parenting behaviors and attitudes. Studies have demonstrated the influence of strong, positive bonding by parents on how they speak to their infants (Ringler et al., 1975), how healthy the infant stays (O'Connor et al., 1977; Pollitt & Gilmore, 1977), and how responsive mother and father are to the infant's signals (Klaus & Kennell, 1976). Most theorists agree that the infant, when sufficiently mature (usually during the second six months of life), will select responsive, salient individuals to whom to become attached (e.g., Ainsworth, 1973; Bowlby, 1958; Cairns, 1966; Schaffer & Emerson, 1964). Thus, the early attachment of parent to newborn facilitates later attachment of infant to parent.

Some neonatal characteristics tend to be maintained perhaps even into adulthood (e.g., activity level and social orientation). The behavioral, temperamental, and personality characteristics that do remain stable over time may do so because they in part shape the environment that nourishes them. The longer a characteristic is unmodified, the less easily it can be changed, and some characteristics are indeed traceable to the earliest days of life.

Costly longitudinal studies such as that reported by Kagan and Moss

(1962) are required to determine the long-range significance of the early postpartum period on the social development of both infant and parents. Theory suggests that early interactions are important for later development. Indeed, developmental psychologists have long suspected that, as Freud claimed, the child is the father of the man—and, furthermore, that the newborn may be the father of the child.

## SUMMARY

The social interaction of the neonate with his or her parents has been the focus of an enormous amount of theoretical speculation and empirical effort in the 1970s. A bidirectional model wherein parent and infant share control of social interaction has guided recent research.

The social world of the neonate is influenced by infant characteristics present before delivery. These include the physical appearance of the infant, the infant's gender, and some infant behavioral predispositions.

Maternal activities during pregnancy such as the use of drugs can alter subsequent social interactive patterns between parent and newborn. Maternal behavior patterns, age, and experience also predict her level of responsiveness to her offspring.

The neonate is an efficient learner who develops primitive but effective social skills quite rapidly. From the moment of birth, the newborn is equipped to become an active participant in the family's social environment.

Parents respond in stereotypic ways to the birth of a child and to the subsequent social signals he or she emits. There may exist a sensitive period for parents after the child is born during which they are most likely to become strongly attached to the infant if allowed extended contact with him or her. The delivery setting advocated by Leboyer (1976) seems especially suited to the quick establishment of the parental bond with the newborn.

## RECOMMENDATIONS

Based on the present review of the interaction of parents and their newborn infants, several recommendations are offered.

Hospitals and other facilities that provide maternal health care should alter any present policies that do not permit extended contact between the neonate and his or her parents. Given the possibility that a sensitive period does exist, the contact should not only be extensive, but it should begin immediately after birth. Although in a small minority of cases certain health considerations may suggest a change, the benefits of early parent-infant interaction must be carefully weighed when any decision to impede such interaction is considered by parents and health care personnel.

Congruent with recommendations that have been made in other chapters (e.g., Chapter 5), the role of good information should be stressed in this context as well. Psychologists, obstetricians, delivery room nurses, and other professionals who work with individuals who are awaiting the birth of a child should provide accurate information to parents on the importance of early parent-infant interactions. Such information will allow the parents a more active and sounder role in making decisions about whether or not to room-in, what type of rooming-in to select, and so on.

For professionals who engage in research on the neonatal period, one area seems of major importance: the intensification of research efforts to determine the long-range consequences of early social events on child and parent. As has been suggested, some possible relationships exist between early interaction patterns and the behaviors measured later in the child's life. Pursuit of the understanding of these specific and long-range relationships seems highly desirable.

Finally, let us make a plea to professionals who deal with parents and newborns. Myths and folklore abound in the area of childrearing procedures and it is only recently that sound investigations of the early neonatal period have been undertaken on a large scale. Professionals should rely on principles that have the strongest empirical support. The history of science in general is full of examples of erroneous assumptions that were carefully guarded by scientific institutions. The emerging information in the study of neonates has provided us with the opportunity to offer to parents clarification and direction based on sound empirical data.

## REFERENCES

AINSWORTH, M. D. S. The development of infant-mother attachment. In B. M. Caldwell and H. N. Ricciutti (eds.), *Review of child development research,* vol. 3. Chicago: University of Chicago Press, 1973.

ALEKSANDROWICZ, M. K., and ALEKSANDROWICZ, D. R. Obstetrical pain-relieving drugs as predictors of infant behavior variability. *Child Development,* 1974, *45,* 935–945.

APPLETON, T., CLIFTON, R., and GOLDBERG, S. The development of behavioral competence in infancy. In F. D. Horowitz (ed.), *Review of child development research,* vol. 4. Chicago: University of Chicago Press, 1975.

BELL, R. Q. A reinterpretation of the direction of effects in studies of socialization. *Psychological Review,* 1968, *75,* 81–95.

———. Stimulus control of parent or caretaker behavior by offspring. *Developmental Psychology,* 1971, *4,* 63–72.

———. Contributions of human infants to caregiving and social interaction. In M. Lewis and L. A. Rosenblum (eds.), *The effect of the infant on its caregiver.* New York: Wiley, 1974.

BELL, R. Q., and COSTELLO, N. S. Three tests for sex differences in tactile sensitivity in the newborn. *Biologia Neonata,* 1964, *7,* 335–347.

BELL, S. M., and AINSWORTH, M. D. S. Infant crying and maternal responsiveness. *Child Development,* 1972, *43,* 1171–1190.

BIRNS, B., BLANK, M., BRIDGER, W. H., and ESCALONA, S. K. Behavioral inhibition in neonates produced by auditory stimuli. *Child Development,* 1965, *36,* 639-645.

BLEHAR, M. C., LIEBERMAN, A. F., and AINSWORTH, M. D. S. Early face-to-face interaction and its relation to later infant-mother attachment. *Child Development,* 1977, *48,* 182-194.

BOWER, T. G. R. *A primer of infant development.* San Francisco: Freeman, 1977.

BOWLBY, J. The nature of the child's tie to his mother. *International Journal of Psychoanalysis,* 1958, *39,* 350-373.

BRAZELTON, T. B. Effect of prenatal drugs on the behavior of the neonate. Paper presented to the American Psychological Association, Miami Beach, 1969.

———. *Neonatal behavioral assessment scale.* Philadelphia: Lippincott, 1973.

BROWN, J. V., and BAKEMAN, R. Antecedents of emotional involvement in mothers of premature and fullterm infants. Paper presented to the Society for Research in Child Development, New Orleans, 1977.

BROWN, J. V., BAKEMAN, R., SNYDER, P. A., FREDRICKSON, W. T., MORGAN, S. T., and HELPER, R. Interactions of black inner-city mothers with their newborn infants. *Child Development,* 1975, *46,* 677-686.

BUDIN, P. *The nursling.* London: Caxton, 1907.

CAIRNS, R. B. Attachment behavior of mammals. *Psychological Review,* 1966, *73,* 409-426.

CALDWELL, B. M. The effects of infant care. In M. L. Hoffman and L. W. Hoffman (eds.), *Review of child development research,* vol. 1. New York: Russell Sage, 1964.

CLARKE-STEWART, K. A. And daddy makes three: the father's impact on mother and young child. *Child Development,* 1978, *49,* 466-478.

CLARREN, S. K., and SMITH, D. W. The fetal alcohol syndrome. *New England Journal of Medicine,* 1978, *298,* 1063-1067.

COHEN, D. J. The crying newborn's accommodation to the nipple. *Child Development,* 1967, *38,* 89-100.

COHEN, S. E., and BECKWITH, L. Caregiving behaviors and early cognitive development as related to ordinal position in preterm infants. *Child Development,* 1977, *48,* 152-157.

CONDON, W. S., and SANDER, L. W. Neonate movement is synchronized with adult speech: interactional participation and language acquisition. *Science,* 1974, *183,* 99-101.

CONWAY, E., and BRACKBILL, Y. Delivery medication and infant outcome: an empirical study. *Monographs of the Society for Research in Child Development,* 1970, *4,* 24-34.

FELDMAN, S. S., and NASH, S. C. Interest in babies during young adulthood. *Child Development,* 1978, *49,* 617-622.

FIELD, T. Effects of early separation, interactive deficits, and experimental manipulations on mother-infant interaction. Paper presented to the Society for Research in Child Development, New Orleans, 1977.

GARN, S. M., SHAW, H. A., and MCCABE, K. D. Effect of maternal smoking on hemoglobins and hemotocrits of the newborn. *American Journal of Clinical Nutrition,* 1978, *31,* 557-558.

GREENBERG, M., ROSENBERG, I., and LIND, J. First mothers rooming-in with their newborns: its impact on the mother. *American Journal of Orthopsychiatry,* 1973, *43,* 783-788.

HARLOW, H. F. *Learning to love.* San Francisco: Albion, 1971.

HOPKINS, J. B., and VIETZE, P. M. Postpartum early and extended contact: quality, quantity, or both? Paper presented to the Society for Research in Child Development, New Orleans, 1977.

HOROWITZ, F. D., ASHTON, J., CULP, R., GADDIS, E., LEVIN, S., and REICHMANN, B. The effects of obstetrical medication on the behavior of Israeli newborn infants and some comparisons with Uruguayan and American infants. *Child Development,* 1977, *48,* 1607–1623.

KAGAN, J., and MOSS, H. A. *Birth to maturity: a study in psychological development.* New York: Wiley, 1962.

KILBRIDE, H. W., JOHNSON, D. L., and STREISSGUTH, A. P. Social class, birth order, and newborn experience. *Child Development,* 1977, *48,* 1686–1688.

KLAUS, M. H., and KENNELL, J. H. *Maternal-infant bonding.* St. Louis: Mosby, 1976.

———. Care of the mother. In E. M. Hetherington and R. D. Parke (eds.), *Contemporary readings in child psychology.* New York: McGraw-Hill, 1977.

KORNER, A. F., CHUCK, B., and DONTCHOS, S. Organismic determinants of spontaneous oral behavior in neonates. *Child Development,* 1968, *39,* 1145–1157.

KORNER, A. F., and GROBSTEIN, R. Visual alertness as related to soothing in neonates: implications for maternal stimulation and early deprivation. *Child Development,* 1966, *37,* 867–876.

LEBOYER, F. *Birth without violence.* New York: Knopf, 1976.

LEIFER, A. D., LEIDERMAN, P. H., BARNETT, C. R., and WILLIAMS, J. A. Effects of mother-infant separation on maternal attachment behavior. *Child Development,* 1972, *43,* 1203–1218.

LESSEN-FIRESTONE, J. K. Maternal attitudes and mother-infant interaction: patterns of reciprocal influence. Paper presented to the Society for Research in Child Development, New Orleans, 1977.

LEWIS, M. Infants' responses to facial stimuli during the first year of life. *Developmental Psychology,* 1969, *1,* 75–86.

LIPSITT, L. P., KAYE, H., and BOSACK, T. Enhancement of neonatal sucking through reinforcement. *Journal of Experimental Child Psychology,* 1966, *4,* 163–168.

LITTLE, R. E., and STREISSGUTH, A. P. Drinking during pregnancy in alcoholic women. *Alcoholism: Clinical and Experimental Research,* 1978, *2,* 179–183.

LOTT, D. F., and ROSENBLATT, J. S. Development of maternal responsiveness during pregnancy in the laboratory rat. In M. Foss (ed.), *Determinants of infant behavior,* vol. 4. London: Methuen, 1969.

MOSS, H. A. Sex, age, and state as determinants of mother-infant interaction. *Merrill-Palmer Quarterly,* 1969, *13,* 19–37.

MOSS, H. A., and ROBSON, K. S. Maternal influences in early social visual behavior. *Child Development,* 1968, *39,* 401–408.

MOSS, H. A., RYDER, R. G., and ROBSON, K. S. The relationship between preparental variables assessed at the newlywed stage and later maternal behaviors. Paper presented to the Society for Research in Child Development, New York, 1967.

NEWTON, N., and NEWTON, M. Mothers' reactions to their newborn babies. *Journal of the American Medical Association,* 1962, *181,* 206.

O'CONNOR, S. M., VIETZE, P. M., HOPKINS, J. B., and ALTEMEIER, W. A. Postpartum extended maternal-infant contact: subsequent mothering and child health. Paper presented to the Society for Research in Child Development, New Orleans, 1977.

OSOFSKY, J. D., and O'CONNELL, E. J. Patterning of newborn behavior in an urban population. *Child Development,* 1977, *48,* 532–536.

PARKE, R. D., and COLLMER, C. W. Child abuse: an interdisciplinary analysis.

In E. M. Hetherington (ed.), *Review of child development research,* vol. 5. Chicago: University of Chicago Press, 1975.

PARKE, R. D., and O'LEARY, S. E. Family interaction in the newborn period: some findings, some observations, and some unresolved issues. In K. Riegal and J. Meacham (eds.), *The developing individual in a changing world.* The Hague: Mouton, 1976.

PARKE, R. D., O'LEARY, S. E., and WEST, S. Mother-father-newborn interaction: effects of maternal medication, labor, and sex of infant. *Proceedings of the 80th Annual Convention of the American Psychological Association,* 1972, *7,* 85-86.

PARKE, R. D., and SAWIN, D. B. Father-infant interaction in the newborn period: a re-evaluation of some current myths. Paper presented to the American Psychological Association, Chicago, 1975.

PEDERSEN, F. A., ANDERSON, B. J., and CAIN, R. L. An approach to understanding linkages between parent-infant and spouse relationships. Paper presented to the Society for Research in Child Development, New Orleans, 1977.

PHILLIPS, S., KING, S., and DUBOIS, L. Spontaneous activities of female versus male newborns. *Child Development,* 1978, *49,* 590–597.

POLLITT, E., and GILMORE, M. Early mother-infant interaction and somatic growth. Paper presented to the Society for Research in Child Development, New Orleans, 1977.

REBELSKY, F., and HANKS, C. Fathers' verbal interaction with infants in the first three months of life. *Child Development,* 1971, *42,* 63-68.

RHEINGOLD, H. L. The development of social behavior in the human infant. *Monographs of the Society for Research in Child Development,* 1966, *31,* 1-17.

RINGLER, N. M., KENNELL, J. H., JARVELLA, R., NAVOJOSKY, B. J., and KLAUS, M. H. Mother-to-child speech at two years: effects of early postnatal contact. *Journal of Pediatrics,* 1975, *86,* 141-144.

RINGLER, N., TRAUSE, M. A., KLAUS, M. H., and KENNELL, J. H. The effects of extra postpartum contact and maternal speech patterns on children's IQs, speech, and language comprehension at five. *Child Development,* 1978, *49,* 862-865.

RUFF, H. A., and HALTON, A. Is there directed reaching in the human neonate? *Developmental Psychology,* 1978, *14,* 425–426.

ST. CLAIR, K. L. Neonatal assessment procedures: a historical review. *Child Development,* 1978, *49,* 280–292.

SCARR, S. Genetic factors in activity motivation. *Child Development,* 1966, *37,* 663-673.

———. Social introversion-extraversion as a heritable response. *Child Development,* 1969, *40,* 823-832.

SCHAFFER, H. R., and EMERSON, P. E. The development of social attachments in infancy. *Monographs of the Society for Research in Child Development,* 1964, *29,* No. 3.

STAAB, R. J., and LYNCH, V. D. Cannabis induced teratogenesis in the CF1 mouse. *Pharmacologist,* 1977, *19,* 179.

STRAUSS, M. E., LESSEN-FIRESTONE, J. K., STARR, R. H., and OSTREA, E. M. Behavior of narcotics-addicted newborns. *Child Development,* 1975, *46,* 887-893.

THOMAN, E. B., KORNER, A. F., and BEASON-WILLIAMS, L. Modification of responsiveness to maternal vocalization in the neonate. *Child Development,* 1977, *48,* 563-569.

WALTERS, C. E. Prediction of postnatal development from fetal activity. *Child Development,* 1965, *36,* 801-808.

WELLER, G. M., and BELL, R. Q. Basal skin conductance and neonatal state. *Child Development,* 1965, *36,* 647–657.

WICKELGREN, L. W. Convergence in the human newborn. *Journal of Experimental Child Psychology,* 1967, *5,* 74–85.

WILSON, A. L. A predictive analysis of early parental attachment behavior. Paper presented to the Society for Research in Child Development, New Orleans, 1977.

# PART III

# CONTRACEPTION AND CHANGE IN THE REPRODUCTIVE SYSTEM

# Chapter 8

# Psychological Dimensions in Controlling Conception

CONTRACEPTION PROVIDES FREEDOM to choose. Couples are able to have a mutually satisfying sexual relationship without serious risk of pregnancy. Use of contraception techniques allows for family planning, with couples now able to limit family size or to specify time intervals between offspring.

Sophistication in the technology of controlling conception has progressed more rapidly than developments in associated human values. Although highly practical and effective methods of contraception exist, significant portions of the sexually active population are poorly informed about them, do not have ready access to them, have conflicting attitudes and emotions concerning their use, encounter social and cultural values incongruent with their use, or experience contraceptive failure. Reflecting existing work, our discussion in this chapter will emphasize factors associated with the occurrence of unwanted pregnancy and with poor fertility management among sexually active single persons. For the most part, women have been the focus of investigations and theorizing. We include in our discussion consideration of men wherever data permit.

## EXTENT AND SCOPE OF THE PROBLEM

Research on unwanted pregnancy and birth has documented the personal and social costs of contraceptive failure. The population boom and the cost of overpopulation are generally accepted as social problems of considerable magnitude (Hardin, 1974; Jaffe and Dryfoos, 1975; Pohlman, 1969). The medical, psychological, and social costs for women of mandatory motherhood have been well documented (Furstenberg, 1976; Rainwater, 1960, 1965). Available data suggest that illegitimate children fare poorly in later life (David, 1973; Dytrych et al., 1975; Forssman & Thuwe, 1966). The longer term effects of abortion on the individual have yet to be firmly established (Leach, 1977; Shusterman, 1976). Thus, it is generally conceded that fertility management and family planning serve both the individual and society.

Family planning agencies abound and it is the goal of these agencies to provide contraceptive services and family planning assistance to those who cannot afford or who do not choose to use such private services. It has been estimated that in 1972 more than 2.6 million women were served by such agencies (Jaffe, Dryfoos, & Corey, 1973). By 1973, organized family planning programs were serving more than 3 million women (Weinburg, 1974). A massive attempt has been made to make contraceptive technology available to those who want it, and there is evidence that a sizable sector of the population is utilizing these services. Although there has been a fairly steady decline in marital fertility over the past eight years, there has been a concomitant rise in the rate of illegitimate births, particularly among teenagers (Morris, 1974). It has been estimated that in 1971, there were 416,127 illegitimate births in the United States. On the basis of studies done in California it has been asserted that this rate has continued to rise (Sklar & Berkov, 1974); moreover, at least 745,000 legal abortions were performed in the United States in 1973. By 1974, that figure rose to over 900,000 (Tietze, Jaffe, & Dryfoos, 1975). In spite of the availability of contraception, a huge number of problem pregnancies and unwanted pregnancies occur each year. Most of these appear to involve single women in their teens and twenties.

A host of studies have documented recent increases in sexual activity among single individuals. Zelnik and Kantner (1977) reported a pair of well-conducted, national, probability sample surveys of women between the ages of 15 and 19. They found that 35% of those interviewed in 1976 had experienced sexual intercourse, as compared with 27% in 1971 (an increase of approximately 30%). Such increases occurred for both blacks and whites and at all ages studied. In 1976, 18% of the 15 year olds and 55% of the 19 year olds sampled were sexually experienced. Furthermore, the median age of first intercourse went down from 16.5 in 1971 to 16.2 years of age in 1976. These surveys did not reveal any marked changes in the frequency of sexual intercourse among sexually experienced teenagers. The overall pattern of increased prevalance of sexual experience makes the possibility of unwanted pregnancy even greater.

## Contraceptive Practices

Within recent years, a number of investigations have explored the sexual and contraceptive practices of various sectors of the society. Random samples of teenagers across the nation, clients seeking assistance from family planning centers or prenatal care clinics, and university students have received particular attention. Such descriptive studies help to clarify existing fertility management behavior.

Three of the major factors associated with contraceptive practices appear to be the age of the person, the pattern of sexual behavior, and the nature of the relationship between the sexual partners. These three variables tend to be correlated, with older persons more likely to be involved in more stable relationships that include ongoing sexual activity. Consequently, determining the separate contribution of each of these factors is often impossible.

McCance and Hall (1972) mailed questionnaires to all female undergraduate students at Aberdeen University and obtained a response rate of 90%. Forty-four percent of the respondents had experienced sexual intercourse, and of those having sexual intercourse during the past six weeks, 39% had had intercourse without using any contraception. On the occasion of first intercourse, 53% reported not using any form of contraception.

Similar findings in university populations have been reported by Cole, Beighton, and Jones (1975) and by Fujita, Wagner, and Prior (1971). The latter researchers found that 54% of males and 42% of females who were sexually active did not consistently use contraception. In a survey of 509 undergraduates at a Canadian university, Munz, Carson, Brock, Bell, Kleinman, Robert, and Simon (1976) found higher rates of contraceptive use, with 90.4% of sexually active respondents described as usually using effective contraception and 79% as always using effective methods.

Furstenberg, Masnick, and Ricketts (1972) examined the contraceptive behavior of a group of adolescent women during the three years following the birth of a first child. Only slightly over half of the women who had begun to use contraception (predominantly the pill) continued to use it one year postpartum. Many of these gave absence of sexual intercourse or highly infrequent sexual intercourse as the reason for nonuse. Evans, Selstad, and Welcher (1976) studied 333 single teenage women seeking assistance for pregnancy related matters (i.e., pregnancy test, abortion, or prenatal care). At the initial interview, those in the abortion and negative pregnancy test groups attributed their not having used birth control to not having intercourse often and therefore not anticipating getting pregnant. At a follow-up interview six months after resolution of the current pregnancy or suspected pregnancy, the largest proportion not practicing birth control said that they were not having intercourse regularly with anyone.

Zelnik and Kantner (1977), in their 1971 and 1976 national surveys of unmarried women between 15 and 19 years of age, found significant changes in contraceptive practive over this time period. In 1971, most sexually experienced individuals used some contraception at some time, but at last intercourse fewer than half were protected. A sharp increase was observed in the number of women who always used contraception from the 1971 to the 1976 sample. Similarly, the percentages protected at last intercourse rose from 42% to 58% for blacks and from 45% to 65% for whites. Those under 17 years of age in 1976 were more likely to have used contraception at last intercourse than those over 17 years of age in the 1971 sample. It should also be noted that the category of women who had never used a contraceptive method also increased, though by only nine percentage points. Furthermore, they found that infrequent intercourse was associated with discontinuance of oral contraceptives or of the intrauterine device (IUD). About two-thirds of the sexually experienced but inactive women continued to take oral contraceptives. About one-third of those whose most recent method was the pill and who had not had intercourse in the past four weeks stopped using the pill, whereas only approximately one-sixth of the women who were sexually active during that period discontinued pill use.

Whelan (1974) reviewed the research literature on the regularity of contraceptive use, approaching the phenomenon from the standpoint of compliance with medical regimes. She cited the findings of Laurie and Korba (1972) that among a large sample of Puerto Rican and U.S. women, one or more tablets were omitted in 14% of birth control pill cycles. Rovinsky (1964) noted that at least 3.1% of women taking oral contraceptives were not following the directions on the package. With respect to vaginal methods of contraception, Whelan (1974) also summarized studies showing striking rates of noncompliance. Pearl (1934) found that 17% of married white women who had experienced one pregnancy were using contraception intermittently for reasons other than a desire for subsequent pregnancy. Chesler (1961) observed that 33% of South African women who relied on the diaphragm for contraception did not use it regularly. Finally, Dingle and Tietze (1963) reported that among their sample of 728 users of foams, tablets, jellies alone, and diaphragm with spermicide, 25% acknowledged irregular use.

## Contraceptive Methods Used

With respect to methods of contraception, although various kinds of oral contraceptives and IUDs have apparently become highly popular among married individuals, these techniques appear less widespread among sexually active nonmarried persons. Studies reporting on the popularity of contraceptive methods practiced by single individuals have identified withdrawal, rhythm, and condoms as the most popular means of birth control, followed by douche, spermicides, and diaphragm (Finkel & Finkel, 1975; Fujita, Wagner, & Prior, 1971; McCance & Hall, 1972). Zelnik and Kantner (1977) observed a change in popularity of various birth control methods between their 1971 sample and their 1976 sample of adolescent women. Use of the pill and IUD showed sharp increases in popularity among those practicing birth control while methods such as condoms, douche, and withdrawal declined.

Research summarized in McCary (1978) and in Whelan (1974) has clearly indicated that the methods most popular among single persons are least effective. Although use of any established method is superior to nothing, failure rates of 33% for rhythm and 39% for douche (Ryder, 1973) are striking. Potential explanations for this pattern of choice focus on the medical supervision necessary for the pill and IUD (the most effective methods), in contrast to the less effective methods, which are available over the counter (e.g., condom, spermicide), and completely private methods such as withdrawal and rhythm (Furstenberg, 1976; Goldsmith et al., 1972). In the latter study, evidence was also obtained that suggested that a greater acceptance of one's sexuality and more active planning characterized single women who took the daily positive action necessary for oral contraception. Finally, from a cost-benefit perspective, significant side effects may be encountered with the use of birth control pills. Protection in infrequent, sporadic sexual intercourse may not seem worth these side effects.

In sum, it would seem that a substantial proportion of sexually active single persons have used some form of contraception although often only on an intermittent basis. Intermittent use seems to be associated with the frequency of sexual activity and the nature of the relationship between the sexual partners. Methods used emphasize procedures that are specific to the sexual episode and can be implemented at that time despite the lesser reliability of these techniques. Public acknowledgment of sexual intent appears to be an underlying factor operating against the use of the more effective, but medically supervised, procedures.

## MAJOR PERSPECTIVES REGARDING UNWANTED PREGNANCY

Although there is a sizable body of sociological literature concerned with population analysis, there is a relatively small body of psychological and sociological literature concerned with the causes and consequences of fertility and with fertility management behavior. Sociology has looked at population analysis primarily in terms of formal demography, e.g., statistical study of human populations with reference to size and density, distribution and vital statistics, as well as population theory, politics, and characteristics. It has not concerned itself with the dynamics of individual behavior or the ways in which a particular social setting influences an individual's behavior (Fawcett, 1970; Freeman, 1976; Pohlman, 1966, 1969). Freeman (1976) noted that although there has been a surge of research in the past decade, few empirical studies have looked at psychological variables in a systematic way and progress in answering crucial research questions in the area of the psychology of fertility management has been limited.

Among researchers concerned with psychological explanations for fertility, there are two traditional perspectives—contraceptive ignorance and intrapsychic conflict. Recently, there has been some concern for looking at psychosocial factors as intervening variables, attempting to explain how the social setting influences and motivates individuals.

### Contraceptive Ignorance

Fundamental to the contraceptive ignorance perspective is the assumption that a lack of knowledge concerning contraceptive methods and/or lack of availability of contraception are primary causes of unwanted pregnancy (Bumpass & Westoff, 1970). Research and theory within this tradition have stressed fertility management behavior as a function of demographic factors such as age, race, and religion.

The idea that contraceptive ignorance is largely responsible for a major portion of unwanted pregnancy dates from the early part of this century. At that time, information regarding contraceptive measures was banned as obscene by federal state laws. McCary (1978) has provided a good summary of recent historical developments regarding legal changes in the area of contraception. He noted that laws prohibiting the mailing, transporting, or giving of contraceptive devices or information perpetuated contraceptive ignorance. Margaret Sanger, in the early part of this century, began to challenge these laws. The federal law and 22 similar state laws, were eventually ruled unconstitutional. According to McCary (1978), the last of these was overturned in 1966.

The Princeton study (Westoff et al., 1961, 1963) focused on variables in three categories: sociocultural environment, personal social orientation toward various aspects of life situation, and selected personality characteristics. As in the earlier studies, however, no significant associations between psychological variables and fertility were identified. Fawcett's (1970) explanation of this fact suggested that the relevant psychological variables either were not chosen or were inadequately measured.

## KNOWLEDGE OF REPRODUCTION AND CONTRACEPTION

The idea that prevalence and efficacy of contraceptive practices rest on adequate knowledge of human reproduction and contraception seems fundamental. Certainly, no contraceptive can be employed without at least technical know-how. Whether increases in knowledge beyond such a minimum is positively associated with improved contraceptive practice is the more significant underlying issue.

Munz et al. (1976), in their study of undergraduates at a Canadian university, developed a test of reproductive and contraceptive knowledge. They defined inadequate knowledge as scores lower than one standard deviation below the mean for a group of second-year medical students who had completed courses in human reproduction and human sexuality. In this study, 66.6% of the males and 65.8% of the females demonstrated an adequate level of knowledge. Overall, 79.8% of sexually active individuals showed adequate knowledge. No significant relationship was found between adequacy of knowledge and age of the individual.

Reichelt and Werley (1975) assessed the overall level of knowledge of 1,327 clients of a family practice clinic (88% were women and the mean age was 16.3). Within a more general questionnaire, they included their own 39-item test of knowledge of birth control and reproductive functioning. The response options included a "don't know" alternative. They found that scale scores were higher for those who were sexually experienced as compared to those who were inexperienced; higher for those using some form of birth control than for those not using any form of birth control, and higher for females than for males. They also found that scores increased with age, education, and socioeconomic level. A majority could correctly answer only two out of the six questions dealing with the pill. One-half of the respondents answered incorrectly the question "Do rubbers break easily?" This item was the only one for which the number of incorrect responses was greater than the number of "don't know" responses. Forty-nine percent to 61% responded correctly to items dealing with withdrawal, rhythm, and douche. One in four did not know when the most fertile part of the menstrual cycle occurs.

Reichelt and Werley noted that as a mandatory part of services from the family planning clinic serving their sample, an educational session with a counselor was required. In their study, women selecting oral contraception had to return in 10 weeks for additional supplies, thus allowing an evaluation of the effectiveness of the educational session for this subsample. They observed that this subsample was similar to the overall sample in the initial level of knowledge. They found a significant increase in total score, as well as substantial increases in the proportion answering most items correctly. One exception to this trend was noted: almost half continued to believe that rubbers break easily and an additional 20% still responded with "don't know" to the question.

Goldsmith, Gabrielson, Gabrielson, Matthews, and Potts (1972) evaluated the sexual knowledge of a group of single women under 17 years of age seeking assistance from family planning centers. Two hundred ten were never-pregnant women seeking contraceptive aid, an additional 100 women were seeking an abortion, and 67 were pregnant women who were carrying unwanted pregnancies to term and living at maternity homes. Between 10 and 30% of the women in each group endorsed the following myths, with the contraceptive group having the lower percentage in each instance: (1) most teenage boys need sex regularly or they will just about go crazy; (2) no birth control can be trusted if it is meant for (fated) a girl to get pregnant; (3) if a boy pulls out before climax, the girl is likely to get pregnant (negative answer is viewed as significant); (4) if you douche right away after intercourse, you are less likely to get pregnant.

Finkel and Finkel (1975) examined the contraceptive knowledge of a sample of 421 high school students with a mean age of 16.3 and approximately evenly divided among black, Hispanic, and white males. Possible scores ranged from zero to six, with six representing greatest knowledge. A score of four or more was obtained by 58%; just over one-fourth scored three; and 15% obtained a score of one or two. There did not appear to be significant variations in knowledge across ethnic groups and knowledge did not increase with age. A score of four or better was obtained by 60% of those having already attended a mandatory hygiene class; among those having not yet attended, only 47% obtained a score of four or better.

One element of contraceptive knowledge receiving particular attention involves the likelihood of becoming pregnant across the menstrual cycle. Zelnik and Kantner (1977) reported that in their 1971 national sample of never-married teenage women, fewer than two in five knew when the period of greatest risk occurs during the menstrual cycle. Only 16% of blacks and 40% of whites demonstrated correct knowledge, with knowledge being associated with age and sexual experience for whites but not for blacks. Their results in the 1976 survey were quite comparable, with only slight increases in the proportion demonstrating such knowledge. These findings appear consistent with those reported by other investigators (Evans, Selstad, & Welcher, 1976).

Presser (1977) has argued that findings concerning knowledge of period of greatest risk tend to be overestimates because of correct guessing on multiple choices. She interviewed a sample of 408 women between 15 and 29 years of age who had just given birth to a first child. Approximately one year later, 358 (88%) were reinterviewed. Only 33% gave the correct response on both occasions; a greater proportion of whites than blacks were knowledgeable; and knowledge appeared to be positively related to age.

A number of studies have reported findings that cast doubt on the role of contraceptive and reproductive ignorance in unwanted pregnancy. Luker (1975) found that 86% of abortion clients she interviewed had used contraception effectively at some time in their lives, and over half of these had used prescription methods. Kane, Lachenbruch, Lipton, and Baram (1973) found that the pregnant women in their study reported knowing where to obtain contraception and did not appear to view the obtaining of it as a problem. Over 90% had an accurate knowledge of at least three forms of contraception, as well as a reasonably good idea of the relative efficacy of different methods. Similar findings were reported by Furstenberg (1976). Munz et al. (1976) concluded that among their sample of undergraduates at a Canadian university, those who risked unwanted pregnancy did so in spite of adequate knowledge. Fujita and associates (1971) reported good factual knowledge within their undergraduate sample, viewing the continued use of rhythm as evidence of a rift between knowledge and behavior in this group.

Goldsmith et al. (1972) concluded, from their comparisons of never-pregnant teenage women seeking contraception and those seeking assistance for an unwanted pregnancy, that acceptance of sexuality was a more important correlate of birth control than was sexual knowledge, education, or religion. The work of Kane and associates (Kane, Moan, & Bolling, 1974; Kane et al., 1973) has supported the notion that for a significant proportion of unwanted pregnancies, motivational factors, rather than lack of knowledge, play the major role.

Perhaps the most commonly identified reason for single individuals not using some form of contraception is that intercourse was not anticipated. Contraceptive preparedness may mean premeditation of sexual intercourse, and such premeditation may enhance the moral unacceptability of sexual activity. Bauman (1971) surveyed a random sample of 100 male and 100 female never-married undergraduates. Bauman found that 22 of the 37 men and 16 of the 29 women having intercourse without contraceptive protection said that sexual intercourse had not been anticipated on that occasion. Similar findings for sexually active college students have been reported by Beard (1973) and by Cole and co-workers (1975).

Goldsmith et al. (1972) studied women under 17 years of age seeking assistance from family planning centers (for contraceptive advice, abortion, or maternity care). They examined the reasons for not using birth control measures. The four most common explanations given were (1) fear of being hassled, (2) "pregnancy couldn't happen to me," (3) "deep down, I might want to get pregnant," and (4) "I wouldn't have intercourse." Women who chose to carry an unplanned pregnancy to term in the study by Evans, Selstad, and Welcher (1976) were likely to indicate the following reasons for not using contraceptive measures: (1) they had not objected so much to becoming pregnant and (2) they had not anticipated the need for birth control.

In sum, it would seem that substantial differences exist across different sectors of the community in adequacy of practical contraceptive and sexual knowledge and that ignorance and misconceptions can significantly increase the risk of unwanted pregnancy; however, knowledge alone is not a sufficient remedy. Individuals reasonably well informed are still apt to engage in intercourse under conditions that risk conception. Not anticipating intercourse and viewing contraception as implying premeditation of sex are reasons frequently given for poor fertility management. In the next sections, we will examine some of the intrapsychic and interpersonal factors offered in studies as potential explanations for failure to practice contraception.

## Personality Factors

Studies focusing on personality factors associated with controlling conception have traditionally adopted a psychodynamic orientation, focusing on the potential role of unconscious conflicts. More recently, some studies have begun to evaluate stable personality characteristics as correlates of contraceptive practice; however, the psychodynamic perspective has dominated thinking within this realm.

The intrapsychic conflict approach asserts that women get pregnant because they experience psychological resistance to using birth control. This school of thought is highly influenced by psychoanalytic theory. Deutsch (1945) saw the problem pregnancy as motivated by the need to resolve Oedipal conflicts. Devereux (1960) pointed to self-punitive impulses and masochism as unconscious causes of inadequate contraception. Blaine (1967) cited the cause as conflicted sexual identity and the need to prove femininity. Lidz (1970) has focused on a variety of factors, including possible conflicts over infertility, the possibility that pregnancy provides a way of proving oneself and demonstrating potency, the possibility that contraceptives were used only because of the financial cost of having a baby or to please a mate, thus generating frustration or unhappiness, and the possibility that for the lonely, depressed, deprived woman pregnancy and a child is a way of satisfying her own emptiness. It should be noted that the successful user of contraceptives does not fare much better in Lidz's view. In general, such a woman is believed to be one who either has several children or feels finished with childbearing, who fears pregnancy for any number of neurotic reasons, or who would rather be a man.

Lehfeldt (1971) pointed to psychological factors in what he called the syndrome of willful exposure to unwanted pregnancy. He clarified that he used "willful" in the Freudian sense, i.e., that this syndrome is neither rational nor conscious but represents an unconscious emotional need for pregnancy arising from psychological factors originating in either or both of the partners.

Sandberg and Jacobs (1971) suggested 14 potential categories of reasons for the misuse or rejection of contraception. They noted that the same behavior (lack of effective contraception) may have a variety of motivational bases. Their speculative categories included denial of risk, shame, embarrassment and guilt associated with sex, masochism, severe depression, sexual identity conflicts, and interpersonal manipulativeness. They summarized their views by suggesting that the personality constellation that will fail most consistently characterizes the "immature, dependent self punishing individual who has a feeling of low self esteem and who has little, if any, desire to control his or her life" (p. 237) Also characteristic of such an individual would be the "inability to assume responsibility, to control impulses, to appreciate long range goals, and develop good sexual adjustment" (p. 237).

Abernethy (1974) suggested a set of personality and background factors that predispose a woman to risk unwanted pregnancy. These included (1) not liking her own mother or finding that she is not an adequate role model, (2) liking her father better than her mother and consciously excluding the mother from family relationships, (3) hostility in the parental marriage, (4) failure to have satisfying relationships with other women, and (5) low self-esteem compensated by self-defeating attempts to feel sexually sought after.

Abernethy, Robbins, Abernethy, Grunebaum, and Weiss (1975) examined their hypotheses through the use of a specially constructed projective technique in which persons were asked to make up stories in response to a series of pictures that could be seen as depicting various family configurations. Responses from 85 women, aged 15 to 45, who were inpatients at two Massachusetts state mental hospitals, were scored for personality and background factors thought to relate to risk of unwanted pregnancy. The scoring was done by four independent judges using specially developed scoring instructions that emphasized hypothesized family elements. Classifications of high, intermediate, or low risk for unwanted pregnancy, based on the responses to this projective technique, were compared to a criterion measure based on self-reported behavior, e.g., whether a woman regularly had sexual intercourse without contraception or did not use contraception on the last occasion of intercourse. Analysis revealed a reliable relationship between these two measures, lending some credibility to the hypothesized psychological functioning of at least some women at risk for unwanted pregnancy. Although such findings are of interest, limitations of the study should be kept clearly in mind. Abernethy et al. observed that generalizability of findings for women in a psychiatric hospital to nonpsychiatric populations is a significant concern. Also, the overall importance of these findings rests on the utility of projective techniques in the study of personality as a whole. In recent years, this general relationship has been questioned.

In general, studies on intrapsychic factors are speculative rather than empirical in nature. For the most part, conclusions are drawn on the basis of the writer's clinical experience with a relatively small and often skewed sample. Most pregnant women do not choose to see a psychiatrist or psychologist, and those who do may well be choosing to do so because they are troubled rather than because they are pregnant. It would seem fallacious to attempt to generalize to a broader population from such samples. Perhaps these studies are most valuable in helping therapists identify some of the factors characteristic of pregnant women who are in therapy.

In addition to difficulties in sampling, the intrapsychically oriented studies tend to focus on the individual in isolation from the social context in which she is acting. Consequently, the prescriptive, preventive, or remedial approach suggests therapy for the individual to help her in overcoming internal resistance to using birth control effectively. Such an orientation may be valuable for women who are already troubled and at risk for unwanted pregnancy; however, this solution is highly impractical and inefficient from the standpoint of family planning agencies. Finally, these studies tend to be highly moralistic in tone and demeaning to women in that they depict problem pregnancy clients as neurotic and deviant.

Some empirical studies have challenged this view. Lynch (1973) found no psychological differences between abortion clients and nonpregnant women on several scales, including Rotter's Locus of Control Scale (measuring the extent to which a person believes she is in control of what happens versus the extent to which she believes that what happens is controlled by external events), Berger's Self-Acceptance Scale, and a five-item scale pertaining to female reproductive activity.

Other studies have examined personality correlates specifically in relation to contraceptive practices. Lundy (1972) administered objective measures of self-esteem, dogmatism, and locus of control to 282 sexually active, unmarried female undergraduates. Lundy used self-reports to divide this group into those who used effective contraception and those who did not. Contraceptive users were found to be significantly lower on the dogmatism scale and significantly closer to the internalized end of the locus of control scale; however, the two groups did not differ reliably with respect to self-esteem. Comparable findings with regard to locus of control were reported by MacDonald (1970). In this study, unmarried female undergraduates scoring in the upper and the lower 27% of a distribution of locus of control scores were compared. Significantly more of the sexually active females scoring toward the internalized end of the scale practiced contraception than did sexually active females scoring toward the externalized end of the scale. The two groups did not differ with respect to proportion having premarital intercourse, number of sexual partners, or time of first intercourse.

Langer (1976) obtained findings that tend to contradict the work of psychoanalytic theorists who view unconscious conflicts and disturbances in sexual gender identity as related to motivation for premarital pregnancy and/or nonuse of contraception. She attempted to determine whether pregnancy is motivated, and if so, to assess the personality factors that might account for such motivation. The factors she explored were (1) motivation for motherhood, using a Thematic Apperception Test based instrument she developed, (2) gender identity, using the Franck Drawing Completion Test, (3) femininity, using the femininity scale of the California Psychological Inventory, and (4) sex role style, using a nine-item questionnaire related to an assertiveness dimension of personal style (McClelland & Watt, 1968). The sample consisted of 129 sexually active college women who were recruited through a psychology class. The only statistically reliable difference Langer found was between contraceptors and noncontraceptors on the sex role style questionnaire. Women who used contraceptives were significantly more assertive than women who were not using contraceptives. In her interpretation of this finding, she pointed out that more traditionally feminine women tie sexuality to reproductivity; thus, the nonuse or inconsistent use of contraception may well be an attempt to place themselves in situations whereby those expectations could be met. It demands a certain amount of assertiveness for women (especially single women in temporary relationships) to obtain and use contraception. Langer made no attempt to explain such role style differences in terms of social or cultural meanings of contraception and pregnancy.

## Sexual Acceptance and Sexual Guilt

One area of personality functioning of obvious importance is sexuality. Development from childhood through adolescence and into adulthood typically necessitates the incorporation of a burgeoning sexuality into one's self-concept. Conflicting social expectations and values often make development in this area difficult. Effective contraception involves a personal, and at times public, acknowledgment of one's sexuality. Consequently, it seems likely that acceptance of sexuality would be associated with more effective contraception.

Goldsmith et al. (1972), in their study of single women under 17 years of age seeking assistance from family planning centers, found that sexual acceptance was positively associated with effective contraception. They observed that never-pregnant women seeking contraception showed less anxiety about masturbation than did women seeking an abortion or women carrying an unwanted pregnancy to term. Furthermore, the group seeking contraception showed the highest acceptance of premarital intercourse. They also rated mutuality of sexual enjoyment as a reason for sex more often than did other groups, and they were more likely to give a rating of "extremely" whereas the pregnant groups were more likely to give a rating of "somewhat" with respect to the enjoyableness of sexual intercourse. Finally, the pregnant women were more likely to have had only one sexual partner in the past than were the women seeking contraception.

Congruent findings were reported by Cole and associates (1975) in their study of undergraduate women. They found that the longer the current relationship between sexual partners, the greater the proportion of women who were using good contraceptive techniques. A strong relationship was also observed between parental discussion and knowledge of daughter's sexual behavior, on the one hand, and good contraceptive practice, on the other. As in the study by Goldsmith et al. (1972), women experiencing a pregnancy were somewhat more likely to have had only one sexual partner in the past than those who were not pregnant but were using contraception. Reiss, Banwart, and Foreman (1975) hypothesized that using contraception effectively would depend on a sexual life-style. Among a sample of 482 undergraduate females, they found a positive relationship between seeking contraceptive assistance and endorsement of sexual choice for the individual, self-assurance, and degree of commitment to the sexual partner.

Lindemann (1975) hypothesized that the degree of commitment to sex would be associated with the type of contraception employed. This line of reasoning would suggest a progression from no contraception through methods that can be implemented at the time of intercourse to medical methods, which are a persistent part of the individual's functioning, e.g., oral contraceptives.

Zelnik and Kantner (1977) reasoned that the distribution of methods of contraception at first intercourse would differ from the distribution at last intercourse. In their national sample of women 15–19 years of age, they found that the most recent occasion showed somewhat more reliance on birth control pills and the IUD and less condom use than did the first intercourse. They reported that among those surveyed in 1976, a surprising number used oral contraceptives or an IUD initially, especially black teenagers. Half of those in their sample who reported having had sex only once did not use any contraception and among those who did use some method, the condom was most common. Those persons in their sample who had had sex more often and who used contraception on the first occasion were likely to continue using conventional methods such as condoms, foams, and spermacides. Individuals who delayed adoption of contraception were likely to begin with medical techniques such as the birth control pill. Interestingly, the difference in quality of method between those who delayed adoption of a method (initially had intercourse without contraception) and those who did not was a matter of age at first use of contraception or previous experience with pregnancy. They noted that this line of reasoning, however, did not account for persons who never used contraception but who had had intercourse more than once.

Feelings of guilt or shame associated with sexuality have often been identified as factors hindering effective contraception. Clearly, in the analysis of misuse and rejection of contraception, Sandberg and Jacobs (1971) pointed to guilt and shame as prominent factors. They noted that use of contraception often increases the visibility of one's sexual behavior and such visibility may be the basis of shame, especially for single persons. Guilt, they speculated, may be associated with sex as a source of sensual pleasure rather than a means of procreation. Kane et al. (1974) interviewed all the residents of four maternity homes. They found guilt over sexual activity to be a prominent reason in not using effective contraception. Many expressed fears of being found out by parents. The attitude that preparation for sexual activity implies promiscuity was also frequently expressed. Kane et al. (1973) found that for 40% of a group seeking abortion, guilt and fear of discovery were associated with the conscious planning of sexual activity. An additional 15% reported conscious feelings of guilt about the use of contraception on a systematic basis. Sitkin (1974) reported that the women in his study evidenced strong disapproval of sex, viewing the pleasure seeking aspects as irregular or illegitimate.

In a systematic study of the relationship between guilt and contraceptive practice, Upchurch (1978) administered Mosher's Forced Choice Scale of Sexual Guilt and a questionnaire dealing with sexual behavior and contraceptive practices to 74 female and 39 male undergraduates. Guilt scores were found to be higher among those who had not had sexual intercourse than among those who reported frequent sexual activity. Sexually active individuals were divided, based on guilt scores, into thirds for females and males separately. The upper and lower thirds were used in subsequent analyses. Eighty-one percent and 54% of low guilt females and males, respectively, had had intercourse within the past week, and 37% and 66.6% of high guilt females and males, respectively, had had sexual intercourse during the same period. Ninety-two percent of the low guilt sexually active women had used a contraceptive measure. Among the high guilt sexually active females, 67% had used a contraceptive measure—a statistically reliable difference. The mean guilt score for females using contraception was 130; for females not using contraception, it was 147. The mean guilt level for those using oral contraception as the method of contraception was 126; for those females using the condom as the method of contraception, the mean guilt score was 176. Contraceptive practices did not appear to vary significantly with guilt scores for males.

In summary, the contribution of personality factors to the nonuse of effective contraception appears mixed. On the one hand, a number of intrapsychic motivational forces have emerged from clinical studies and theorizing; however, these are probably most relevant for psychologically troubled women who become pregnant. In studies that used more objective measures of personality factors, some evidence has been accrued that suggests that for women, more effective contraceptive practice is associated with assertiveness, lack of dogmatism, and the belief that one has control over what happens (internal locus of control). The most prominent personality area appears to be the individual's orientation toward sexuality. Acceptance of her own sexuality appears to be positively related to effective contraception whereas sexual guilt and shame appear to operate against such effective use.

## Psychosocial Orientation to Fertility Management

One of the challenges facing psychology in the field of family planning is explaining the relationship among the individual's social environment, emotional status, and motivation for contraception (Fawcett, 1970). What psychosocial explanations can account both for differentials in fertility and fertility related behavior identified in surveys and for shifts over time in such variables (Fawcett, 1970)?

Rainwater's (1960, 1965) work represents an early attempt to develop an accurate social explanation for fertility differentials shown to exist across social classes. Rainwater considered the relationship of class, race, and religion to fertility, viewing conjugal role organization and marital sexual relationship, family size preference, and motivation for contraception as the intervening variables that affect fertility management. He observed that successful fertility management was related to a variety of factors including the degree of conjugal mutuality as opposed to conjugal role segregation, as well as the degree to which the wife was accepting of her own sexuality and the couple enjoyed a mutually gratifying sexual relationship. His findings led him to conclude that lower-class women are typically less accepting of their own sexuality than more middle-class women and that lower-class marriages tend to be characterized by less mutually gratifying sexual relationships than their middle-class counterparts. He found, moreover, that lower-class marriages are more often characterized by role segregated conjugal relationships than middle-class marriages. He noted that family size preferences are, to some extent, related to a woman's dependence on the role of mothering for her self-esteem, pointing out that lower-class women tend to have fewer social and intellectual interests outside the home and see fewer alternatives to the wife and mother role than do middle-class women. He suggested that effective contraceptive behavior is linked not only to the ease with which couples are able to communicate about sex and family planning (which is related to the degree of mutuality of sexual enjoyment) but also to the ability of the woman to assert herself. The findings of this study, focusing as it did on marital and social roles as intervening variables, clearly lend support to the notion that the female sex role is somehow related to effective fertility management behavior.

Several other studies have focused on the relationship of the female role and fertility management behavior. Having reviewed the literature, Scanzoni and McMurry (1972) concluded that perception of female role does influence both family size desired and contraceptive effectiveness. They noted that less traditional women will tend to stay single longer, report a desire for fewer children, and actually have a smaller family. Scanzoni (1976) examined the relationship of gender roles within marriage to "birth orientation" (desires and intentions with regard to family size). "Gender status" (wife as junior partner or as equal partner) was found to have a significant effect on birth orientation and expected success of contraception. When only those households were considered in which wives worked full time, the strength of these relationships increased markedly. Kar (1971), in a survey of 209 married couples, found that early acceptance of contraception (before first pregnancy) was positively correlated with level of striving, social optimism, value orientation, and future orientation.

Presser (1974), relying on her assessment of young mothers in the New York area, attributed ill-timed early motherhood to a combination of factors including knowledge and motivation. In discussing the implications of her findings, she indicated that she believed the way to strengthen motivation to seek out and use contraception would be to change the early socialization patterns of women. She suggested that the relationship between the roles of women and the timing of first birth and subsequent fertility should be evaluated in future research. Showing agreement with this line of reasoning, Klerman (1975) speculated that (1) narrow definitions of female roles, (2) a discrepancy between actual sexual practices and moralistic societal attitudes toward sexual practices, and (3) a lack of societal purpose and meaningful work all contribute to adolescent pregnancy.

Miller (1973) explored the relationship between female role orientation and reproductive behavior. He hypothesized that a woman's perception of the adult female role is linked in a significant way to her reproductive career. Miller surveyed the responses of 967 never-married and just married women and women who had recently become mothers. His findings, though somewhat inconclusive, suggest that in general a more modern orientation toward the female role is associated with later marriage and a desire for fewer children. His data suggest that women with a modern orientation tend to be somewhat more effective contraceptive users.

Irons (1978), in her doctoral dissertation, assessed attitudes toward the rights and roles of women, psychological androgyny (extent to which an individual shows behaviors sex typed as appropriate for males as well as behaviors sex-typed as appropriate for females), perceived work options for women, and attitudes toward sex and abortion among four groups of women: successful contraceptors, first time abortion seekers, repeat abortion clients, and women carrying unwanted pregnancies to term. The latter group showed a significantly more traditional orientation than did the other three groups, which did not differ reliably from each other. Compatible findings were reported by Goldsmith et al. (1972) in their comparison of contraceptors, abortion clients, and residents of a maternity home. Contraceptors were found to be significantly more oriented toward higher education and postponement of marriage than the pregnancy groups. The authors reported that the contraceptive group appeared to be more achievement oriented and to plan their lives more than the other groups.

Luker's (1975) work dealt with contraceptive risk taking. She argued that such behavior is the result of a dynamic decisionmaking process employed by women who are both informed and rational. In a preliminary study, she used open-ended, relatively unstructured interviews with abortion seeking women. From these interviews emerged categories that Luker later called the cost of contraception and the benefit of pregnancy. She hypothesized that women who choose to take contraceptive risks choose to do so on the basis of a cost-benefit analysis comparing the costs and benefits of using birth control against the costs and benefits of possible pregnancy. She argued that the decision is typically a rational one, given the societal context within which they make this decision.

The social and cultural costs of using contraception cited by Luker are directly related to the definition of female sex roles and norms for role appropriate behavior. In order to use birth control effectively, a woman must break a good number of the rules of traditional sex typed behavior. A woman who uses contraception is taking an active stance in managing her own sexuality and fertility. She is acknowledging that she is planning intercourse and actively dissociating her sexuality from her reproductive functions. This is norm breaking behavior, especially for single women; moreover, the benefits identified in Luker's study are sex role specific. Pregnancy is viewed as a way of proving womanliness. Pregnancy is a way of establishing that one is capable of producing children and thus that one is capable of performing the primary function for which this society rewards women.

In summary, although empirical data are meager, existing evidence suggests that psychosocial factors contribute significantly to fertility management behavior. In particular, perceptions and beliefs concerning sex role appropriate behavior of women appear influential in fertility management. Better contraceptive management apparently is related to more modern, liberal views of women. Previously reviewed findings that related better contraceptive management to assertiveness and acceptance of sexuality would seem to be highly consistent with the overall conclusion.

## OVERVIEW

From the present review of research and theorizing, it would seem that a number of factors contribute to the effectiveness with which individuals practice contraception. Frequency and regularity of sexual intercourse, nature of the relationship between the sexual partners, age of the individual, knowledge concerning sexual and contraceptive functions, motivational factors, acceptance of sexuality, sexual guilt, internalized locus of control, dogmatism, and more modern orientation toward women and women's role have all been found to be associated with contraceptive behavior. At least some of the relationships might be incorporated by a view of sexuality as an internal personality disposition.

Conflicting cultural and personal values and beliefs at times interfere with an individual's viewing his sexual behavior and sexual feeling as a stable part of himself. The perception of oneself as a sexual person might be expected to be influenced by a number of factors including the physical development of the person from childhood to adulthood, sexual experience, role expectations, and social roles regarding sex.

Within the field of social psychology, a body of theory and research under the heading of attribution theory deals with the way in which individuals develop causal explanations for behavior (e.g., whether a particular act of violence is viewed as a product of external, situational forces or as a product of the internal disposition of the actor). The process responsible for the naive observer's explanation of behavior is the prime concern. Such factors as the social desirability of behavior, the frequency of behavior over time, and the consistency of behavior across different situations (Harvey, Ickes, & Kidd, 1976) have been shown to influence whether a given behavior is viewed as the product of external, situational factors or the product of internal, personality factors.

In the present context we are suggesting that to the extent that sexual occurrences are viewed as a product of situational or external factors, contraceptive practices will be haphazard or nonexistent; however, when sexual occurrences are viewed as a product of internal characteristics of the individual, adequacy of contraception will improve—assuming conception is not desired and assuming the necessary level of contraceptive knowledge exists.

Thus, the occasional sexual encounter of the single adolescent would be more congruent with viewing the sexual experience as a product of situational factors. As noted, a common reason given for not using contraception is "I was not planning on having sex." As the relationship between sexual partners becomes more stable, sexual activity is also likely to become more frequent and consistent, leading to improved contraceptive practices; however, from an attributional perspective, the sexual behavior may be attributed to the specific relationship rather than to the disposition of the individual. Termination of the relationship would be associated with termination of contraception. Such reasoning was offered by Furstenberg, Masnick, and Ricketts (1972) and by Zelnik and Kantner (1977) for the discontinuance of birth control pills. A related finding of some interest is that women seeking an abortion or carrying an unwanted pregnancy to term were more likely to have had only one sexual partner than were never-pregnant single women seeking contraceptive assistance (Goldsmith et al., 1972). Sexual behavior with more than one partner would discourage attribution to a specific relationship and thus likely enhance viewing sexuality as part of the individual.

As pointed out in our section on psychosocial factors, women have traditionally been viewed as passive sexual objects, tolerating sexual encounters as part of their marital responsibilities. If such a view is associated with adult women in marital relationships, the sexual behavior of single adolescent women would be seen as even more counternormative and socially undesirable. Personal responsibility for such behavior might be disclaimed. The findings relevant to the role of sexual guilt and shame are particularly pertinent. It would seem reasonable to expect that the strength of such feelings would be positively related to unwillingness to accept sexual behavior and feelings as a part of one's personality. Consequently, increases in sexual guilt would be associated with less adequate contraceptive practices. A particularly relevant finding for this line of reasoning is the association between locus of control and adequacy of contraceptive practices. As observed by MacDonald (1970), better contraceptive practices were associated with individuals scoring toward the internalized end of the dimension. Overall, internalizers are seen as believing that they have more control over their lives than externalizers feel. It seems reasonable to expect that this general belief orientation would also characterize their view of sexual occurrences.

The positive relationship between assertiveness and contraceptive behavior is also consistent. Obtaining and utilizing the most effective methods of birth control necessitates public acknowledgment of sexual behavior and sexual intent. Public visibility of such counternormative behavior would be expected to lead to attributions to personal dispositions. A behavioral style of assertiveness would seem an important correlate of such public acknowledgment.

Although active recognition and acceptance of sexual behavior and feelings for women might be counternormative on a general level, such interpretations might be expected to vary with some demographic and personal factors. For instance, feminist attitudes toward women and a more egalitarian view of marriage might well be attitudinal correlates of positive norms regarding female sexuality. Decreases in the degree to which sexual behavior and feelings of women are viewed as counternormative would be expected to facilitate viewing such elements as a part of the individual and thus improve contraceptive practices.

The finding that acceptance of sexuality is strongly related to contraceptive behavior is especially meaningful. These findings and formulations would appear most closely tied to the present line of reasoning. The degree to which a person is committed to sexual behavior as described by Lindemann (1975) and by Zelnik and Kantner (1977), the perception of sexual choice as studied by Reiss, Banwart, and Foreman (1975), and the view of sexual occurrences as highly pleasurable as identified by Goldsmith et al. (1972) would seem consistent with the view of one's sexual behavior and feelings as a part of personality makeup. Viewing oneself as a sexual person provides a basis for acknowledging potential sexual encounters and taking steps for adequate preparation.

Variations in contraceptive behavior may be influenced by a variety of factors. The same contraceptive behavior may result from differing combinations of causal factors. For instance, unprotected intercourse may occur because of ignorance concerning the period of greatest risk during the menstrual cycle, because of severe depression or self-punitive attitudes, because of a desire to demonstrate femininity, because of a role definition of women as passive sexual objects, or because of a system of norms that operates against viewing sexual behavior and feelings as a stable part of the individual. It seems unlikely that at our present stage of knowledge one overall theoretical structure can be developed that would integrate satisfactorily the full range of potential causes. We believe, however, that the attributional perspective adds a powerful conceptual tool toward this end.

## REFERENCES

ABERNETHY, V. Illegitimate conception among teenagers. *American Journal of Public Health,* 1974, *64,* 662–665.

ABERNETHY, V., ROBBINS, D., ABERNETHY, G. L., GRUNEBAUM, H., and WEISS, J. L. Identification of women at risk for unwanted pregnancy. *American Journal of Psychiatry,* 1975, *132,* 10.

BARKER-MANTAGU, G. Psychiatric illness after hysterectomy. *British Medical Journal,* 1968, *2,* 91–95.

BAUMAN, K. E. Selected aspects of the contraceptive practices of unmarried university students. *Medical Aspects of Human Sexuality,* 1971, *8,* 76–89.

BEARD, R. M. A study of selected factors in the use/nonuse of contraception. *Dissertation Abstracts International,* 1973, *34*-B, 2124–2125.

BLAINE, G. B. Sex among teenagers. *Medical Aspects of Human Sexuality,* 1967, *2,* 11.

BUMPASS, L. L., and WESTOFF, C. F. *The later years of childbearing.* Princeton: Princeton University Press, 1970.

CHESLER, J. The use of contraceptive diaphragms: a follow-up study of a group of women. *South African Medical Journal,* 1961, *35,* 323–324.

COLE, J. B., BEIGHTON, F. C. L., and JONES, I. H. Contraceptive practice and unplanned pregnancy among single university students. *British Medical Journal,* 1975, *4,* 217–219.

DAVID, H. P. Abortion trends in European socialist countries and in the U.S. *American Journal of Orthopsychiatry,* 1973, *43,* 376–383.

DEUTSCH, H. *The psychology of woman.* Vol. 2: *Motherhood.* New York: Grune & Stratton, 1945.

DEVEREUX, G. The female castration complex and its repercussions in modesty, appearance, and courtship etiquette. *Ameri Imago,* 1960, *17,* 3–19.

DINGLE, J. T., and TIETZE, C. Comparative study of three contraceptive methods: vaginal foam tablets, jelly alone, and diaphragm with jelly or cream. *American Journal of Obstetrics and Gynecology,* 1963, *85,* 1012–1022.

DOWNS, P. E. Intrafamily decision making in family planning. *Journal of Business Research,* 1977, *5,* 63–74.

DYTRYCH, Z., MATEJCEK, Z., SCHULLER, V., DAVID, H. P., and FREIDMAN, H. L. Children born to women denied abortion. *Family Planning Perspectives,* 1975, *7,* 165–171.

EVANS, J. R., SELSTAD, G., and WELCHER, W. H. Teenagers: fertility-control behavior and attitudes before and after abortion, childbearing, or negative pregnancy test. *Family Planning Perspectives,* 1976, *8,* 192–200.

FAWCETT, J. *Psychology and population.* New York: Population Council, 1970.

FINKEL, M. L., and FINKEL, D. J. Sexual and contraceptive knowledge, attitudes, and behavior of male adolescents. *Family Planning Perspectives,* 1975, *7,* 256–260.

FORSSMAN, H., and THUWE, I. One hundred and twenty children born after application for therapeutic abortion refused. *Acta Psychiatrica Scandinavica,* 1966, *42,* 71–88.

FREEDMAN, R., WHELPTON, P. K., and CAMPBELL, A. A. *Family planning, sterility, and population growth.* New York: McGraw-Hill, 1959.

FREEMAN, E. W. Abortion: beyond rhetoric to access. *Social Work,* 1976, *21,* 483–486.

FUJITA, B. N., WAGNER, N. N., and PRIOR, R. J. Contraceptive use among single college students. *American Journal of Obstetrics and Gynecology,* 1971, *109,* 787–793.

FURSTENBERG, F. F., JR. *Unplanned parenthood.* New York: Free Press, 1976.

FURSTENBERG, F. F., JR., GORDIS, L., and MARKOWITZ, M. Birth control knowledge and attitudes among unmarried pregnant adolescents: a preliminary report. *Journal of Marriage and the Family,* 1969, *31,* 34–42.

FURSTENBERG, F. F., JR., and MASNICK, G. S., and RICKETTS, S. A. How can family planning programs delay repeat teenage pregnancies? *Family Planning Perspectives,* 1972, *4,* 54.

GOLDSMITH, S., GABRIELSON, M. O., GABRIELSON, I., MATTHEWS, V., and POTTS, L. Teenagers, sex, and contraception. *Family Planning Perspectives,* 1972, *4,* 32–38.

HARDIN, G. *Mandatory motherhood: the true meaning of "right to life."* Boston: Beacon, 1974.

HARVEY, J. H., ICKES, W. J., and KIDD, R. F. (EDS.). *New directions in attribution research,* vol. 1. Hillsdale: LEA, 1976.

HASS, P. H. Wanted and unwanted pregnancies: a fertility decision-making model. *Journal of Social Issues,* 1974, *4,* 30.

IRONS, E. The causes of unwanted pregnancy: a psychological study from a feminist perspective. *Dissertation Abstracts International,* 1978, *38*-A, 5354.

JAFFE, F. S., and DRYFOOS, J. G. Fertility control services for adolescents: access and utilization. *Family Planning Perspectives,* 1975, *7,* 167–175.

JAFFE, F. S., DRYFOOS, J. G., and COREY, M. Organized family-planning programs in the U.S., 1968–1972. *Family Planning Perspectives,* 1973, *5,* 73.

KANE, F. J., JR., LACHENBRUCH P., LIPTON, M. A., and BARAM, D. Motivational factors in abortion patients. *American Journal of Psychiatry,* 1973, *130,* 290–293.

KANE, F. J., MOAN, C. A., and BOLLING, B. Motivational factors in pregnant adolescents. *Diseases of the Nervous System,* 1974, *35,* 131–134.

KAR, S. B. Individual aspirations as related to early and late acceptance of contraception. *Journal of Social Psychology,* 1971, *83,* 235–245.

KLEIN, L. Early teenage pregnancy, contraception, and repeat pregnancy. American Journal of Obstetrics and Gynecology, 1974, *120,* 249–255.

KLERMAN, L. V. Adolescent pregnancy: need for new policies and new programs. *Journal of School Health,* 1975, *45,* 263–267.

LANGER, G. B. Pregnancy and motherhood motivation in unmarried women: some intrapsychic, interpersonal, and behavioral factors. *Dissertation Abstracts International,* 1976, *36,* 4694.

LAURIE, R., and KORBA, V. Fertility control with continuous microdose Norgestrel. *Journal of Reproductive Medicine,* 1972, *8,* 165–168.

LEACH, J. Repeat abortion patient. *Family Planning Perspectives,* 1977, *9,* 37–39.

LEHFELDT, H. Psychology of contraceptive failure. *Medical Aspects of Human Sexuality,* 1971, *5,* 68–77.

LIDZ, T. The family as the developmental setting. In E. J. Anthony and C. Koupernik (eds.), *The child in his family.* New York: Wiley, 1970.

LINDEMANN, C. *Birth control and unmarried young women.* New York: Springer, 1975.

LUKER, K. *Taking chances: abortion and the decision not to contracept.* Berkeley: University of California Press, 1975.

LUNDY, J. R. Some personality correlates of contraceptive use among unmarried female college students. *Journal of Psychology,* 1972, *80,* 9–14.

LYNCH, M. Psychological study of premaritally pregnant college women seeking abortion. *Dissertation Abstracts International,* 1973, *33,* 6085.

MACDONALD, A. P. Internal-external locus of control and the practice of birth control. *Psychological Reports,* 1970, *27,* 206.

MCCANCE, C., and HALL, D. J. Sexual behavior and contraceptive practice of unmarried female undergraduates at Aberdeen University. *British Medical Journal,* 1972, *2,* 694–700.

MCCARY, J. L. *McCary's human sexuality.* New York: Van Nostrand, 1978.

MCCLELLAND, D. C., and WATT, N. F. Sex-role alienation in schizophrenia. *Journal of Abnormal Psychology,* 1968, *73,* 226–239.

MILLER, W. B. Psychological vulnerability to unwanted pregnancy. *Family Planning Perspectives,* 1973, *5,* 199.

MORRIS, L. Estimating the need for family planning sources among unwed teenagers. *Family Planning Perspectives,* 1974, *6,* 91.

MORRIS, N. M., and SISON, B. S. Correlates of female powerlessness: parity, methods of birth control, and pregnancy. *Journal of Marriage and the Family,* 1974, *36,* 708–712.

MUNZ, D., CARSON, S., BROCK, B., BELL, L., KLEINMAN, I., ROBERT, M., and SIMON, J. Contraceptive knowledge and practice among undergraduates at a Canadian university. *American Journal of Obstetrics and Gynecology,* 1976, *124,* 499–503.

PEARL, R. Contraception and fertility in 4945 married women. *Human Biology,* 1934, *6,* 355–401.

POHLMAN, E. H. Birth control: independent and dependent variable for psychological research. *American Psychologist,* 1966, *21,* 967–970.

———. *Psychology of birth planning.* Cambridge: Schenkman, 1969.

PRESSER, H. Early motherhood: ignorance or bliss? *Family Planning Perspectives,* 1974, *6,* 8–14.

———. Guessing and misinformation about pregnancy risk among urban mothers. *Family Planning Perspectives,* 1977, *9,* 111–116.

RAINWATER, L. *And the poor get children.* Chicago: Quadrangle, 1960.

———. *Family design: marital sexuality, family size, and contraception.* Chicago: Aldine, 1965.

REICHELT, P. A., and WERLEY, H. H. Contraception, abortion, and venereal disease: teenagers' knowledge and the effect of education. *Family Planning Perspectives,* 1975, *7,* 83–88.

REISS, I. L., BANWART, A., and FOREMAN, H. Premarital contraceptive usage: a study and some theoretical explorations. *Journal of Marriage and the Family,* 1975, *37,* 619–629.

ROVINSKY, J. Clinical effectiveness of a low-dose progestin-estrogen combination. *Journal of Obstetrics and Gynecology,* 1964, *23,* 840–850.

———. Abortion in New York City: preliminary experience with a permissive statute. *Journal of Obstetrics and Gynecology,* 1971, *38,* 333.

———. Abortion recidivism. *Journal of Obstetrics and Gynecology,* 1972, *39,* 649.

RYDER, W. B. Contraceptive failure in the United States. *Family Planning Perspectives,* 1973, *5,* 133.

SANDBERG E. and JACOBS R. Psychology of the misuse and rejection of contraception. *American Journal of Obstetrics and Gynecology,* 1971, *110,* 227–242.

SCANZONI, J. Gender roles and the process of fertility control. *Journal of Marriage and the Family,* 1976, *38,* 677–691.

SCANZONI, J., and MCMURRY, M. Continuities in the explanation of fertility control. *Journal of Marriage and the Family,* 1972, *34,* 315–322.

SCHNEIDER, S. M., and THOMPSON, D. S. Repeat aborters. *American Journal of Obstetrics and Gynecology,* 1976, *126,* 316-320.

SHATKIN, E. P. Teen-age pregnancy: the family background. *Pediatrics,* 1972, *50,* 167.

SHUSTERMAN, L. R. The psychosocial factors of the abortion experience: a critical review. *Psychology of Women Quarterly,* 1976, *1,* 79-106.

SITKIN, E. M. Measurement of prospective fantasy and other factors in pregnant black teen-age girls. *Dissertation Abstracts International,* 1974, *34,* 4058.

SKLAR, J., and BERKOV, B. Teenage family formation in postwar America. *Family Planning Perspectives,* 1974, *6,* 80-90.

TIETZE, C., JAFFE, F. S., and DRYFOOS, J. G. The unmet need for legal abortion services in the U.S. *Family Planning Perspectives,* 1975, *7,* 197-202.

UPCHURCH, M. L. Sex guilt and contraceptive use. *Journal of Sex Education and Therapy,* 1978, *5:,* 27-195.

WEINBURG, P. C. Psychosexual impact of treatment in female genital cancer. *Journal of Sex and Marital Therapy,* 1974, *1,* 155-157.

WESTOFF, C. F., POTTER, R. G., JR., and SAGI, P. C. *The third child.* Princeton: Princeton University Press, 1963.

WESTOFF, C. F., POTTER, R. G., JR., SAGI, P. G., and MISHLU, E. G. *Family growth in metropolitan America.* Princeton: Princeton University Press, 1961.

WHELAN, F. M. Compliance with contraceptive regimens. *Studies of Family Planning,* 1974, *5,* 349-355.

WHELPTON, P. K., CAMPBELL, A. A., and PATTERSON, J. E. *Fertility and family planning in the United States.* Princeton: Princeton University Press, 1966.

ZELNIK, M., and KANTNER, J. F. Sexual and contraceptive experience of young unmarried women in the United States, 1976 and 1971. *Family Planning Perspectives,* 1977, *9,* 55-71.

# Chapter 9

# Psychological Correlates of Menopause and Climacteric

MENOPAUSE IS THE MOST APPARENT EVENT of the reproductive processes occurring during midlife. The cessation of menstruation demarcates the close of reproductive capacity for women. It is the marker of a major transition within the life cycle. This transition encompasses physiological, psychological, and social events. The present chapter examines current literature dealing with psychological, social, and some physical aspects of menopause and the climacteric.

The normal period of transition in women, and perhaps in men, from having the capacity to reproduce to no longer having that capacity is referred to as the climacteric. Menopause refers specifically to the cessation of menstruation and may be thought of as the counterpart of menarche (Jaszmann, 1976; Utian, 1977). Cope (1976) observed that fertility declines sharply during the four years preceding the menopause, with anovulatory cycles becoming more common. Menstrual cycles become more irregular until they cease altogether.

The last menstruation most often occurs at approximately 51 years of age. Although studies have indicated some variation in the mean age of menopause for particular samples, most report means have clustered around 51 years (Flint, 1976). Jaszmann (1969) mailed a survey to all the women between 40 and 60 years old in a community in the Netherlands. He had a response rate of 71% and found that the age of menopause was normally distributed, with a mean of 51.4 years and a standard deviation of 3.8 years. In this study, age at menopause was found not to be related to age at menarche, number of pregnancies, or age at last pregnancy. Women who had never been married were found to have a statistically earlier mean age at menopause (50.3) than women who were or had been married (mean age of 51.4).

Flint (1976), having made a thorough review of cross-cultural evidence, concluded that age at menopause appears to be related to parity, marital status, abortions, familial pattern, and race; however, overall findings relevant to such factors seemed rather tenuous. She cited reports that diseases such as diabetes, uterine fibroids, cervical polyps, and cancer of the body of the uterus, cervix, and breast are associated with late age of menopause whereas cancer of the ovaries and vulva, pruritus senilis, and hernia are associated with early menopause.

Though empirical findings on the age of menopause appear to be fairly consistent and specific, it seems that women may anticipate menopause much earlier than it usually occurs. McEwan (1973) and Galloway (1975), speaking from their clinical experience, both observed that women in their late thirties and early forties, with a variety of physical symptoms, often asked whether their condition was caused by the "change of life." Such questioning suggests that as a psychological issue, concern about menopause may antedate menopause itself by a considerable period of time.

Lauritzen (1975) noted that menopause is a consequence of the aging of the ovaries; according to him, these are the only endocrine glands that cease to function long before the end of life. Ovarian insufficiency results in estrogen insufficiency. Fedor-Freybergh (1977), in reviewing hormonal changes, observed that the functioning of the corpus luteum diminishes, with decreased steroid hormone production leading to a decrease in feedback inhibition of the hypothalamus, resulting in increased LH (luteinizing hormone) and FSH (follicle stimulating hormone) production. According to Fedor-Freybergh, an increased plasma level of FSH is one of the best hormonal indications of an established climacteric.

Reduction in estrogen production is generally seen as the fundamental hormonal change, though Lauritzen (1975) suggested that menopausal symptoms may result from a relative decrease of estrogen activity on the target tissues rather than from a fall in the absolute level of estrogens. Coope (1976) examined some physical changes correlated with estrogen deficiency. Prominent among these were osteoporosis (or osteopenia), resulting in increased risk of fracture. He also indicated that at menopause, decreased estrogen is associated with a negative nitrogen balance, with muscle being replaced by fibrous tissue. The epidermis thins and subcutaneous fat atrophies, affecting particularly the breasts, which atrophy and lose their shape. Finally, Coope pointed out that estrogen deficiency may be associated with coronary artery disease, noting that in nonsmoking women before menopause, coronary artery disease is extremely rare, whereas, after menopause, the incidence approaches that for men. However, the so-called protective effect of estrogens on coronary artery disease has been seriously questioned (see the section of this chapter that examines side effects of estrogen therapy). Overall, menopause and the attendant changes in hormonal functioning appear to be a landmark in the aging process.

As several authors have pointed out (Cooper, 1976; Cope, 1976), it is only within this century that the average life expectancy of women has exceeded the average age at menopause. For this reason Cope noted that menopause has not been a major social problem until recent times. Van Keep (1976) indicated that approximately 5% of women in the world are between 45 and 54 years old. The number of post-menopausal women continues to rise. Consequently, social, psychological, and physical aspects of such aging have increasing personal and social significance.

The climacteric in men is much less well documented in the research and clinical literatures. Androgen production although gradually decreasing with age, continues in most men until death. Kinsey (1948) found only 25% of American men impotent at 70 years. The mean number of orgasms reported per week dropped from 1.5 at age 55 to between .5 and 1.0 at age 70–not a dramatic change. Henker (1977) reviewed the earlier literature and noted that it is difficult to reconcile the midlife symptoms of men, reported and characterized as a male menopause or climacteric, with an abrupt decline in androgen production. The latter does not seem to occur commonly. However, he described 50 men, between 40 and 60 years of age, selected from a total of nearly 500 men on a psychosomatic service. Their physical complaints included multiple vague symptoms such as chest pain, shortness of breath, hypertension, palpitations, numbness and tingling of extremities, headaches, musculoskeletal pain, gastrointestinal pain, weakness, fatigue, and poor appetite. Sexual inadequacy was described by all. Anxiety was seen in all and depression in 34. Forty-one complained of mild intellectual or memory deficits. He concluded that the male climacteric involves a rather vague syndrome having physical, emotional, and sexual symptoms. The syndrome resulted from a complex interaction of hormonal, situation, physical and psychological factors.

## PROMINENT CLINICAL FEATURES ASSOCIATED WITH MENOPAUSE

Although differences of opinion exist among professionals concerning whether particular symptoms are directly associated with menopause, most seem to view vasomotor symptoms, such as hot flushes and night sweats, as cardinal features. The term "hot flushes," or "hot flashes," refers to a sensation of heat passing through or over the body, with the blush zone (i.e., face, neck, and anterior chest) being most frequently and severely affected. Dewhurst (1976) reviewed some of the existing evidence bearing directly on the frequency and severity of such vasomotor symptoms. He noted, concerning a study conducted by McKinlay and Jefferys (1974) in which 638 women between the ages of 45 and 54 responded to a questionnaire, that 75% of those who had not menstruated during the last 3–12 months reported experiencing hot flushes. Eighty-two percent of the women whose menopause had occurred five years previously reported having had hot flushes for more than a one-year period. Among the women in this study who reported experiencing hot flushes, 48.5% said they felt acute physical discomfort; some had embarrassment also in connection with the hot flushes.

Dewhurst (1976) noted that comparable data were reported by Thompson (1973) in which postmenopausal women in a general practice in Scotland were surveyed. Seventy-four percent of these women reported experiencing hot flushes. Among the 90 patients who reported on the frequency of hot flushes, 49.9% indicated that they occurred daily and 21% said they experienced flushes every few hours. A physician was consulted for relief of such vasomotor symptoms by 45% of the respondents.

Utian (1977), summarizing the views expressed at an international conference on menopausal research, indicated that hot flushes, perspiration, and atrophic vaginitis are probably linked specifically to estrogen deficiency associated with menopause. Many other investigators have described a host of rather nonspecific emotional difficulties experienced by women during this period of life. Kerr (1976), relying on her clinical experience, described the dominant emotional picture in terms of anxiety, depression, tension, and irritability. According to her, there is often a vague sense of internal inadequacy, with a feeling of no longer being able to achieve gratification. Individuals experiencing such distress are likely to complain of involuntary, easily precipitated crying episodes. From her experience, unusual sensitivity to rejection and fear of loneliness may be especially prominent.

Cooper (1976), in discussing some aspects of menopausal distress, observed that the International Health Foundation carried out a major survey in 1969. Two thousand women between the ages of 46 and 55 were sampled in Belgium, France, West Germany, Ireland, Italy, and Great Britain. Within this sample, the most common symptoms were flushes, tiredness, nervousness, sweats, headaches, insomnia, depression, irritability, joint and muscle pain, dizziness, palpitation, and formication. Additionally, these women reported worrying most about depression, faulty memory, obesity, brittle bones, and painful sexual relations.

Jaszmann (1969, 1976), in his survey of women in a community in the Netherlands, grouped respondents on the basis of recent menstrual pattern and looked for differences in symptom picture as a function of these groupings. Group A consisted of women still displaying their regular menstrual pattern and group B consisted of women whose menstrual pattern had been different during the past 12 months in comparison with their preceding pattern. Group C, women whose last menstrual period had occurred sometime before, was subdivided by the length of time since last menstruation. For C1, the last menstruation was 12–15 months earlier; C2, 26–36 months; C3, 37–48 months; C4, 48–60 months; and C5, 5–10 years. Results indicated that symptoms like fatigue, headache, irritability, dizziness, and, to a lesser degree, depression had the highest frequency among group B respondents. Symptoms such as hot flushes, perspiration, formication, and pains in muscles and joints were the most frequent in the early postmenopausal groups (C1 and C2). The Blatt Menopausal Index (BMI) was also highest among women in group C1, probably because of the heavy weighting given symptoms such as hot flushes in this index.

## MENOPAUSE AND PSYCHIATRIC ILLNESS

The climacteric and psychiatric disturbance have long been linked in the thinking of many mental health professionals. The diagnostic category of involutional melacholia (*Diagnostic and Statistical Manual II* of the American Psychiatric Association, 1968) refers specifically to persons who experience an affective psychosis for the first time during the involutional phase of life, presumably including the climacteric.

A number of investigators have begun to challenge the concept of a menopausal psychiatric syndrome (Dominian, 1977; McKinlay and McKinlay, 1973), as well as the notion that menopause directly causes major affective disturbance (Winokur, 1973). Dominian (1977) pointed to the findings of Spicer, Hare, and Slater (1973) that menopause coincides with the age range of peak admissions for depression and commented that these may not be causally related and may have led to a fortuitous connection in the clinical experience of many practitioners.

Winokur (1973) studied 71 women admitted for affective disorders to a psychiatric in-patient unit. Twenty-eight of these women had already passed menopause. He sought to determine whether there is a greater risk for the onset of affective psychosis during menopause (defined, for his purposes, as the three-year interval following the date given by the women for her last menstruation) than during other periods of the life span. Risk was defined as the number of episodes of affective disorder associated with an event divided by the total number of years available for that event. The overall risk for the 71 women was 6%; a 7.1% risk was associated with the menopausal period. This difference did not achieve statistical significance, leading to the conclusion that, within this sample at least, the menopausal period was not linked to the onset of a major affective disorder even among predisposed persons.

Ballinger (1975, 1976a, 1976b) sought to determine whether there is a link between psychiatric symptoms and menopause. Seven hundred sixty women between the ages of 40 and 55, who were patients of six practitioners, were contacted by letter and asked to fill out the General Health Questionnaire (GHQ). This test is a screening instrument for nonpsychotic psychiatric illness. Their scores were examined as a function of menopausal status, chronological age, and presence of vasomotor symptoms. Five hundred thirty-nine of the women returned a completed questionnaire; of these, 155 (28.8%) scored above 12 on the GHQ. This score was viewed as the cutoff for a psychiatrically significant protocol. Menopausal status was defined in terms of four groups: premenopausal, if the women had regular menstrual patterns; menopausal, if there had been three or more missed periods but less than one year of absent menses; postmenopausal, if between one and five years had elapsed since last menstruation; and a final postmenopausal group, if menstruation had ceased more than six years previously. The menopausal group had a significantly higher proportion of women with psychiatric symptoms (by GHQ) than did any of the other groups. When chronological age and menopausal status were combined, the significant rise in psychiatric symptomatology was first seen in the premenopausal women of 45–49 years of age. This increase was maintained over the year of the menopause, followed by a significant reduction in subsequent postmenopausal years. Ballinger speculated that this pattern may reflect biochemical changes antecedent to the cessation of menstruation. Or, it may reflect culturally defined expectations of considerable distress at the time of the menopause, with the subsequent decline in morbidity occurring when such negative expectations are not fulfilled. Interestingly, it has been established for some time (Adamopoulous, 1971; Coble, 1969) that in many women plasma levels of gonadotropins rise significantly two to five years before menopause. Levels of estrogens may or may not be reduced in these women.

Dominian (1977), in his analysis of the evidence concerning the relationship of menopause with psychiatric illness, pointed out that many of the symptoms typically associated with menopause are the same as those found in anxiety states or moderate reactive depressions. This similarity in symptom picture was also identified by Winokur (1973). Aylward (1976), in a study of 596 randomly selected postmenopausal women in whom the period of climacteric amenorrhea ranged from 6 to 28 months, found that 56% of them exhibited prominent features of depression. Within this group, the most common symptoms were inability to make decisions (79%), apathy (65%), irritability (51%), depressive thought content (47%), sleep disturbance (46%), psychomotor retardation (38%), and loss of libido (38%). In conceptualizing such findings, Dominian (1977) identified several alternatives. First, anxiety and depressive states may be physiologically linked to the biochemical changes occurring at menopause; second, such symptoms may arise from life events typical of this period; third, menopause may represent one of several life changes that can independently or in conjunction with other changes give rise to such emotional responses.

Little mention is made of the syndrome of involutional depression (melancholia) in the recent literature. It seems logical that with the increase in life expectancy and in the absolute number of individuals living through the involutional period, involutional depression would assume increasing importance and frequency. However, statistical studies have shown a dramatic decrease in the incidence and prevalence of this condition compared with 25 or more years before. There has been speculation that this may be the result of a real change in the incidence of the illness, or of change in diagnostic practices, or of early therapeutic (particularly psychotropic medication) intervention in those patients who in pre-drug therapy years might have gone on to develop the syndrome. It was never clear that this syndrome was directly related to the climacteric, either in men or in women. Kielholz in 1959 found a peak prevalence in women 50–60 years of age, with onset usually 3–7 years after the menopause. The peak prevalence in men was between 61 and 65 years. These kind of data have suggested and reinforced the common clinical impression that the climacteric in men occurs some 10 years later than in women. Controlled studies examining the possible relationship between the normal climacteric and an involutional depressive syndrome are few. Nikula-Baumann (1971) found that if such a syndrome exists at all, it bears no relationship to the menopause. Her research showed significant changes in adrenal cortical involutional melancholics. However, her study found no significant difference in urinary excretion of estrogens in women melancholics compared with a normal sample.

## PSYCHOLOGICAL AND SOCIAL FACTORS

Most writers view psychological and social factors as significant influences on the way in which women respond to menopause. Negative social attitudes, feelings of diminished femininity, and grief responses to various losses (real and fantasied) are illustrative of the kind of psychosocial variables often included in discussions of this period. Despite the general recognition of the potential importance of such variables, there is a paucity of systematic empirical assessments of their actual contributions. Investigators have instead relied on case histories, clinical impression, extension of psychoanalytic theory, or analysis of cultural content as bases for their speculations. Consequently, in reviewing these ideas, it should be kept in mind that they are suggestive rather than definitive accounts.

The basic assumption of the psychosocial viewpoint was well stated by

McCandless (1964): "While climacteric in women is frequently signaled by the physiological manifestation of ovarian involution, these symptoms tend to focus on, rather than cause, the psychological problems of the climacteric. Emotional difficulties, when they occur, arise from the discontinuity and transition of sociological roles before and after cessation of menses," (p. 489). Such an interpretation emphasizes the psychological significance of the menopause in the context of the life span.

As noted by various authors (Brown, 1976; Dominian, 1977; Fedor-Freybergh, 1977; Galloway, 1975), women between the ages of 45 and 55 are likely to see their children reach adulthood, leave home, get married, and have children of their own. Furthermore, for many women during these years, their own parents become ill and die. Such events produce marked alterations in their social networks. Many of the most important interpersonal relationships (e.g., those between parent and child) across generations are significantly altered. Several authors (e.g., Brown, 1976; Galloway, 1975) have speculated that the psychological impact of such change in the network of interpersonal relationships would depend, to a significant degree, on the psychological assets of the woman, especially the extent to which she has roles outside of housewife and mother. Fedor-Freybergh (1977) noted that the "empty nest syndrome," beginning when children are mature enough to begin leaving home, has been associated with the onset of depression (Humphrey, 1976).

Family theorists have noted that the departure of children is also likely to affect the marital relationship. Completion of childrearing, by definition, involves the end of this activity as one focus of the relationship between wife and husband. It may be necessary for the couple to seek out new areas of mutual interest. Furthermore, as the network of interpersonal relationships changes, the relative importance of the husband-wife relationship may increase, leading to a greater awareness of, or sensitivity to, the quality of the marriage. In such ideas (Galloway, 1975; Dominian, 1977), the wife-mother is seen as taking the psychological brunt of such changes. Sex role stereotypes view women as oriented more toward internal relationships within the family whereas men are seen as oriented primarily toward relationships and activities outside the family (Lidz, 1970). This outside orientation of men is thought of as a stabilizing, moderating influence, diminishing the impact of changes in the family structure.

Although the salience of the marital relationship may heighten for the woman during the climacteric period, strains experienced by the husband may have a negative impact on marital satisfaction. As observed by Brown (1976) and Galloway (1975), men in middle age are likely to experience a plateau in their careers, facing strong competition from younger men. Retirement is a growing reality, and there may be an increasing number of deaths among family, friends, and associates. Physiologic climacteric in men, although poorly documented and understood, may also affect the marriage and the wife. As men begin to feel themselves growing old, whether or not hormonal changes are occurring, there may be a flagging of sexual interest or the development of an orientation toward younger women. Brown (1976) suggested that such issues may lead a husband to focus on events outside his marriage at a time when a wife is looking to that marriage for emotional support, enhancing her fears of being abandoned or unloved. Dominian (1977), in reviewing the limited and often contradictory empirical findings concerning marital satisfaction across the entire life span (Blood & Wolfe, 1960; Bossard & Boll, 1955; Burr, 1970; Deutscher, 1959; Pineo, 1961; Rollins & Feldman, 1970), suggested that a decline in affectionate companionship, with or without deterioration of sexual relations, underlies such marital dissatisfaction.

Numerous investigators (Brown, 1976; Cooper, 1976; Cope, 1976; Van Keep, 1976) have hypothesized that social attitudes and values concerning menopause will substantially affect the psychological distress experienced at this time. Richardson, in a book entitled *Menopause: The Neglected Crisis* (cited in Cope, 1976), argued that the menopause has been seen as a negative event with no importance within the life of a community. Termination of a woman's capacity to reproduce has been viewed as representing an end of her usefulness. Menopause thus is a marker heralding the onset of old age. Cope (1976) noted that according to the Talmud, if a woman misses three periods she is old but if her periods resume she is young again.

The transition through menopause has often been viewed as an undesirable social event. Mead (cited in Cooper, 1976) has described societies in which postmenopausal women are no longer expected to display appropriate feminine behavior. A similar expectation is documented in the writings of some mental health professionals speculating about the psychological significance of the menopause. Osofsky and Seidenberg (1970) identified notable examples. For instance, Deutsch, a well-known psychoanalytic theorist concerned with the psychology of women, in 1945 stated: "The preclimacterium is a time of protest against imminent danger and the menopause itself is a time of disappointment and mortification." She commented further: "The moment the expulsion of the ova from the ovaries ceases, all of the organic processes devoted to the service of the species stop. Woman has ended her existence as a bearer of future life and has reached her natural end—her partial death as a servant of the species." In citing such positions, Osofsky and Seidenberg (1970) pointed out that traditional social values seem to have entailed a view of biology as destiny for women, with their social worth based on reproductive capacity.

However, Van Keep (1976) summarized a discussion at a recent international symposium on menopause, pointing out that the significance of the menopause, and therefore its psychological implications, differs among societies. In the Rahput classes of India menopause is viewed as a positive state and is reported to be associated with few symptoms. Menopausal women are seen as emerging from *purdah* at the end of their childbearing years. They acquire higher status and can move around at will. In this same discussion it was observed that for some Arab women menopause also represents a positive change and that such women evidence less distress than researchers had anticipated. Thus, the emphasis on youth in Western culture may contribute substantially to the distress of women going through menopause.

The frequently documented negative social attitude toward the failure of reproductive capacity through climacteric change (or other cause) is not limited to women. Although history and anecdote reflect the notions that women reach climacteric before men and that barren marriage is woman's fault, they also highlight the loss of virility as a prime source of scorn and ridicule for men. The impotent man could not obtain, or sustain, a young wife and found his standing in the community jeopardized. Notably, the word "impotent," currently used to denote procreative, sexual, or erectile failure in men, derives from the Latin for "not powerful" and continues to this time also to mean weakness in general or even lack of self-control. According to Webster, virile (from the Latin "man") refers to that which "has the qualities of an adult man, specifically capable of procreation." Loss of reproductive capacity thus signals the end of the period of adult manhood and power, which began at the termination of childhood.

In reviewing the psychosocial events characteristic of the climacteric many authors have highlighted the role of loss, both real and symbolic, at this time (Brown, 1976; Cooper, 1976; Dominian, 1977; McEwan, 1973). Loss of children, loss of parents, loss of opportunities, loss of youth, and loss of physical attractiveness are prominent. Cessation of menstruation serves as a social focus on which these changes in life circumstances converge. Loss and depression have long been linked in clinical research and theorizing (Freud, 1917). Depression and anxiety during the climacteric are considered responses to these losses. Social and personal attributes, as well as societal values, that diminish the extent of loss would be expected to be associated with less distress. Although such speculation is widespread, it has not been adequately tested through prospective, systematic empirical studies correlating social and personal attributes with the occurrence or severity of depression at this time of life.

## THE ROLE OF ESTROGEN DEFICIENCY AND ESTROGEN REPLACEMENT

The relationship of estrogen to physical symptoms occurring during the climacteric has been a focus within much of the literature. Reduced plasma estrogen levels associated with the cessation of ovulation and menses have been linked with the concept of an estrogen deficiency syndrome—a constellation of signs and symptoms specifically linked to the decline in estrogen and to the use of estrogen in the treatment of climacteric distress. There appears to be fair agreement that hot flushes, perspiration (particularly in the form of night sweats), and atrophic vaginitis result from lack of estrogen and that estrogen therapy constitutes an effective form of treatment for these symptoms (Coope, 1976; Cope, 1976; Utian, 1977). Lauritzen (1975) identified physical symptoms related to atrophic changes in the vulva, urethra, and bladder and osteoporosis as additional indications for estrogen therapy. Although clinical anecdotes suggest that postmenopausal women often complain of urinary frequency, nocturia, stress incontinence, and dysuria, Osborne (1976) found no significant postmenopausal increase in stress incontinence and urinary frequency in a study of 600 healthy, employed women between 33 and 65 years old. He did find an increase in nocturia (defined as one or more urinations per night) after menopause; 16% of premenopausal women compared with 25% of postmenopausal (this is significant at the 5% level).

Smith (1976) found that of 719 women with urinary frequency and dysuria presenting to a urologist over two years, 292 first developed these symptoms after menopause. His work suggested that estrogens may be helpful in treating these symptoms (especially in combination with urethral dilation) if atrophic vaginitis is also present.

Diffuse loss of bone mass (osteoporosis) with loss of height, kyphosis, and back pain caused by vertebral compression fractures have been associated with menopause since Albright and Reifenstein (1949). Early clinical attempts to treat established postmenopausal osteoporosis with estrogen replacement were disappointing. However, more recent controlled studies (Aitken, 1976) have found that estrogen replacement significantly prevents or retards loss of bone mass if treatment is begun within three years of surgical oophorectomy (castration) in preclimacteric women. However, convincing clinical, longitudinal, controlled studies of the role of estrogens in retarding or reversing symptoms of osteoporosis in normal climacteric or postmenopausal women are not yet available.

Finally, the so-called protective effect of estrogens on the development of coronary artery disease and myocardial infarction needs comment. The incidence of these cardiac difficulties is clearly very much lower in premenopausal women compared with men of the same age. It rises, approaching that of men of the same age, after menopause. However, the assumption that this pattern directly reflects estrogen's action has proven difficult to establish. The infarction rate increases in premenopausal women with other risk factors (such as smoking) given birth control pills. And, attempts to reduce mortality and recurrent infarction by giving estrogen to men with a previous infarct either produce no change (with low doses of estrogen) or actually increase morbidity because of vascular events (with higher doses). The effect of estrogen replacement on arteriosclerotic mortality and morbidity in postmenopausal women has not been adequately established in prospective studies. However, the documented effect of estrogen replacement in elevating blood pressure in some women so treated also suggests caution in predicting estrogen usefulness in reducing cardiovascular deaths in postmenopausal women.

The role of estrogens in the genesis and treatment of psychological symptoms such as depression, anxiety, irritability, insomnia, memory loss, and concentration deficits has been a point of great debate. Jeffcoate (1960) has argued that emotional disturbances are in no way related to hormone changes and therefore such disturbances should not be treated with estrogens. Wilson and Wilson (1963), in contrast, have argued that depression, emotional lability, and irritability reflect estrogen lack and have recommended treatment with estrogens.

Kerr (1976), in examining these issues, cited the work of Neugarten and Kraines (1965) in which 480 women were evaluated, comparing the symptoms reported by menopausal women with those reported by women in other groups. Adolescent women (between 13 and 18 years of age) and menopausal women (aged 45–54) reported the most symptoms. In the latter group women who reported themselves as nonmenopausal had lower symptom scores than those who reported themselves as menopausal. Neugarten and Kraines felt that changes in sex hormones contributed substantially to such symptoms.

Ballinger (1977), in her study of the relationship of psychiatric morbidity and the menopause, examined changes in morbidity as a function of reported vasomotor symptoms. She noted that changes in frequency of vasomotor symptoms were most clearly related to changes in estrogen levels. Among menopausal and immediately postmenopausal women those with evidence of psychiatric disturbance were no more likely to report the presence of hot or cold feelings than were those without evidence of psychiatric disturbance. Among premenopausal women, such vasomotor complaints were much more likely to be made by women with indications of psychiatric disturbance than by those without such indications, though vasomotor complaints overall were infrequent among the premenopausal group. Similarly, for those women who were six or more years postmenopausal, psychiatric status was significantly related to the frequency of complaints of hot or cold feelings. Again, women with significant indications of psychiatric disturbance reported that these symptoms occurred more, or much more often, than usual.

Complementary results were obtained by Jaszmann (1976) in his epidemiological study. Complaints such as fatigue, irritability, headaches, dizziness, and, to a lesser degree, depression had the highest frequency among women whose menstrual pattern had been different during the past 12 months in comparison with their preceding pattern; hot flushes, perspiration, formication, and pain in the muscles and joints were most frequently reported by women in early postmenopause. He viewed the former symptoms as psychosocial manifestations of the beginning of the menopausal transition whereas the latter symptoms were interpreted as evidence of hypothalamic disregulation related to a decrease in endogenous estrogen production.

Though such findings appear neither definitive nor conclusive, they do make suspect the hypothesis of a simple, direct relationship between reduced estrogen levels and onset of emotional distress in the climacteric. However, even without support of such a specific connection, controlled trials of estrogen therapy might still prove replacement therapy beneficial. Fedor-Freybergh (1977) provided an overview of the clinical opinion and empirical work dealing with the effectiveness of estrogen therapy in alleviating menopausal symptoms. He noted that the general impression gained from a series of papers based on subjective evaluations of postmenopausal women taking estrogen was that estrogen considerably improved the mental status of these women (Andor, 1974; Dapunt, 1967; Hauser & Wenner, 1974; Lauritzen, 1971; Radmayr, 1970; Winter, 1967). Fedor-Freybergh (1977) also identified with Lang (1970) a contrasting point of view suggesting that estrogen has only a placebo effect. Early on, Pratt and Thomas (1937) and Segaloff (1949) suggested that placebo, phenobarbital, and bromide are as effective as estrogen therapy in treating menopausal symptoms. In recent years, a number of better controlled studies evaluated estrogen therapy against placebo using double-blind procedures.

Coope (1976) conducted a double-blind crossover study of 30 menopausal women seen in a general medical practice. Thirty-five women began the study, all of whom had at least one symptom included in the Cuperman Menopausal Index. All participants were told that they would be given two preparations during a six-month period—one estrogen and one a harmless, inert tablet. One group was given three 21-day courses of Premarin (conjugated equine estrogens), 1.25 milligrams daily, with a 7-day hiatus between courses. A second group was given placebo following the same pattern. After three months the groups were crossed over. Five patients left before completion of the study. Both groups showed striking improvement in the first three months. Although estrogen produced lower mean scores, the placebo response was also great, and no statistically reliable differences between placebo and estrogen groups emerged. However, after the crossover, those withdrawn from estrogen showed a sudden deterioration, returning to initial levels while those changing from placebo to estrogen evidenced further improvement. With respect to the severity of hot flushes, they found a significant reduction by estrogen as compared with placebo. Although placebo improved this symptom considerably, it was usually necessary to give estrogen to abolish flushes completely. About one-third of the patients showed no improvement with any treatment. These were suffering mostly from weakness, depression, or headaches.

Fedor-Freybergh (1977) assessed estrogen therapy in women who came to an out-patient department of a hospital for treatment of climacteric complaints. Group 1 consisted of 27 premenopausal women reporting irregular menstruation and recent onset of hot flushes, nervousness, anxiety, depression, and sleep disturbance. Treatment consisted of 2 milligrams daily of estradiol for 23 days followed by 1 milligram on days 24 and 27 but placebo on days 25, 26, and 28. On days 13–22 d-norgestrel (a progestational agent) was added. The second group consisted of 25 women who had been amenorrhic for at least 12 months and who were treated with estradiol (the same dose) daily for 28 days. Again d-norgestrel was added as above. The third group consisted of 25 postmenopausal women, divided into two subgroups: in double-blind fashion 13 women (group 3A) received 2 milligrams daily of estradiol for three months while the remaining 12 women (group 3B) received placebo over this period. On self-rating scales of overall clinical improvement, estrogen treated women (groups 1, 2, and 3A) reported feeling better after treatment; a slight deterioration was reported by those receiving placebo. Group 3A (estrogen) showed a decreased neuroticism score and an increased extroversion score on the Eysenck Personality Inventory whereas group 3B (placebo) showed the reverse after the three months of treatment. Estrogen treated groups showed significant (compared to both baseline and placebo) reduction in depression measured by the Hamilton Rating Scale for Depression (HSD). For those on placebo the Sabbatsberg Distress Self-rating Scale and the HSD indicated a small but significant ($p < 0.01$) increase in distress and depression at three months. Compared with placebo, estrogen therapy also significantly improved performance on some tests of cognitive function.

Changes in the Sabbatsberg Sexual Self-rating Scale also correlated with estrogen therapy. Improvements were noted in libido, sexual satisfaction, activity, and fantasy, and orgasm capacity as early as one month into estrogen treatment. A decrease in anxiety (measured by the self-rating scale) was found with estrogen treatment but not with placebo. Finally, improved ability to sleep was reported by all estrogen treated patients. Results of this study need to be interpreted with caution because double-blind procedures existed only for group 3 and because it encompassed a relatively short time period. Interestingly, a final sentence before Fedor-Freybergh's (1977) summary stated that "no negative side effects due to estrogen treatment were reported" (p. 89).

Campbell and Whitehead (1977) reported a pair of especially well designed studies. In each, a double-blind crossover paradigm was followed. In the first, 68 patients with severe symptoms, primarily vasomotor, took part in a four-month study—two months on cyclical Premarin, 1.25 milligrams daily, and two months on daily placebo. In the second, 68 patients with less severe symptoms participated in a 12-month study: 6 months on daily Premarin (same dose) and 6 months of placebo. All participants were either postmenopausal or "had at least 3 months between menses'' (i.e., apparently perimenopausal). Eleven patients left the studies before completion—seven of these were taking placebo and four were taking estrogen at the time. As a check on compliance, urinary excretion of estrogens and vaginal cytology were assessed every two months. These measures documented an increase in urinary estrogens and in vaginal mucosa estrogen effect for all patients participating in an estrogen group.

In the short-term study, compared to pretreatment baselines a significant placebo effect was observed on self-rated vaginal dryness, memory, urinary frequency, youthful skin appearance, and coital satisfaction. However, estrogen was significantly better than placebo in relieving vasomotor symptoms, vaginal dryness, insomnia, irritability, anxiety, urinary frequency, worry about self and aging, headache, memory, good spirits, and optimism. Unfortunately these improvements were reported only in terms of mean scores of groups and without reporting the percentage of patients showing significant improvement in symptoms. Campbell and Whitehead (1977) noted that there appeared to be a ''domino effect,'' with improvement in vasomotor symptoms causing improvement in the large number of predominantly physical symptoms noted above. In those patients who did not suffer from hot flushes, estrogen treatment (compared to placebo) was associated with improvement only in vaginal dryness, poor memory, and anxiety. In the longer term study, placebo effect on vaginal dryness and urinary frequency disappeared over time and the beneficial impact of estrogen on these symptoms was enhanced. Additionally, the effect of estrogen on decreasing complaints of anxiety, vasomotor symptoms, and poor memory was maintained or improved. These authors suggested that the domino effect was not as marked in the long-term study since the patients were selected for less severe vasomotor symptoms compared with patients in the short-term study. Depression (Beck Depression Self-report Inventory) improved significantly in both the estrogen and the placebo group. There was, however, no significant difference in improvement in depression between the estrogen and placebo groups.

Side effects other than vaginal bleeding were frequent while on estrogen (8–21% of patients) and were not uncommon (for example, up to 10% of patients experienced breast tenderness) while on placebo. Breakthrough and withdrawal bleeding while on estrogen occurred in 28–100% of patients depending on how many replacement cycles had been administered and on perimenopausal versus postmenopausal status.

Endometrial hyperplasia occurred in 23% of patients at the end of six months of estrogen therapy but was not found at all after six months of placebo. The authors also cited evidence that either reducing the dose of estrogen (to .625 milligrams Premarin) or adding a progestin (noresthisterone) for 7 days of every 28 days will prevent or reverse the development of such hyperplasia.

Schneider, Brotherton, and Hailes (1977), in a nonblind study treating 20 postmenopausal women with estrogen (conjugated equine estrogens, or CEE) over four weeks, found that improvement in the Beck Depression Self-Report Inventory was related inversely to the severity of the depression. Thus, of 10 patients with Beck depression scores of less than 18, 9 showed improvement. However, of 10 patients with scores of 20 or more, 6 were more depressed after treatment. All women in this latter group of 10 remained within the moderate to severely depressed range and the mean score for the group did not shift toward normal with estrogen treatment. These results suggest that estrogens may improve mild depression associated with, and perhaps secondary to, the physiological symptoms of estrogen deficiency. But, for menopausal women experiencing moderate to severe depression, treating physical symptoms by estrogen replacement may have little or no effect on the depression.

There is increasing evidence that the several different estrogenic preparations currently available have differing therapeutic and side effects. Such variability has been noted in animal studies. The potential clinical importance of this apparent heterogeneity for target symptoms and for side effects in menopausal women is not yet established. It has been suggested that natural estrogens (e.g., conjugated equine preparations) may produce fewer harmful side effects than synthetic preparations. Lozman, Barlow, and Levitt (1971) compared two estrogen preparations, a synthetic (piperazine estrone sulfate, or PES) with naturally occurring compounds (conjugated equine estrogens) in the treatment of menopausal patients. They employed a double-blind crossover paradigm without placebo in 168 patients beginning the study and 131 in the final analysis. Flushes, sweats, headaches, insomnia, depression, and anxiety were the menopausal symptoms reported in pretreatment interviews. Both agents were found to be effective in reducing target symptoms. A greater effect of PES in relieving insomnia was the only statistically reliable difference between the two agents in symptom relief. Vaginal cytology was used as the objective measure of estrogen influence. Although both agents produced improvement when given first and after crossover both maintained the improvement first produced by the other, PES caused statistically significant further improvement when it was the second drug administered. Finally, significantly more of the patients preferred PES to CEE.

A few investigators have attempted to identify the biochemical basis of the effect of estrogen therapy on depression. Noting the similarity of symptoms in menopausal distress and reactive depression, Aylward (1976) has used biochemical findings in studies of depression to hypothesize that decreased free plasma tryptophan is an etiologic factor in menopausal symptoms. In a study of postmenopausal women Aylward found that fasting plasma levels of free tryptophan were significantly lower in depressed than in nondepressed women. Depression (as measured by the Hamilton Rating Scale for Depression) was greater in those with lowest concentrations of free plasma tryptophan. Using double-blind procedures with a placebo control in a small sample, he found that in those treated with estrogen there was a marked increase in plasma estrogen, estradiol, and free plasma tryptophan and an improvement in depression. The placebo treated group did not show significant change in these measures.

Klaiber, Kobayashi, Broverman, and Hall (1971) found that plasma monoamine oxidase activity (MAO) in estrogen deficient women was higher than that found in normal menstruating women. In such deficient women estrogen treatment returned MAO activity to the level found in the preovulatory phase of the menstrual cycle in menstruating women. Looking at the suspected role of MAO activity in some forms of depression, Klaiber, Broverman, Vogel, and Kobayashi (1976) conducted a double-blind study of the effects of estrogen in severely depressed women. He found that estrogen (CEE) significantly alleviated depression as measured by the Hamilton Rating Scale for Depression and reduced the MAO activity of the plasma. Placebo treated patients did not show comparable improvement.

## Side Effects of Estrogen Treatment

In examining the results of estrogen therapy, the demonstrated benefits must be weighed against known adverse effects associated with its use. As yet undetected long-term effects are also cause for concern. The association of diethylstilbesterol treatment in pregnant women with the development of vaginal malignancies in their daughters many years later highlights the need for continued reevaluation of risk-benefit ratio. Campbell and Whitehead (1977), in discussing side effects of estrogen therapy, cited the work of Smith, Prentice, Thompson, and Hermann (1975), Ziel and Finkle (1975), and Mack, Pike, Henderson, Pfeffer, Gerkins, Arthur, and Brown (1976) as suggestive of a link between estrogen therapy and endometrial carcinoma. Campbell and Whitehead criticized this work as being retrospective and poorly documented. In their long-term double-blind study (1977), they found that 7% of patients had endometrial (cystic glandular) hyperplasia at admission to the study. As mentioned, this figure rose to 23% at the end of six months of Premarin (CEE) treatment while no patients had hyperplasia after six months of placebo.

Two recent studies (Antunes et al., 1979; Jick, et al., 1979) have strongly supported an association between endometrial carcinoma and estrogen use. The association is apparently dose and time related and is particularly high with estrogen use of five years or more. Also, both studies found that neither cyclic treatment nor added progestins significantly reduced the risk of such endometrial cancer. Reviewing this and other data, the February-March 1979 issue of the *FDA Drug Bulletin* concluded: "Estrogens are effective . . . for vasomotor symptoms of the menopause and can be used with no known increase in risk for the treatment of this common problem if doses are kept low and the period of treatment is less than one year" (p. 3).

Lauritzen (1976) described a number of clinical conditions in which estrogen therapy is contraindicated. These include severe liver disease, porphyria, recent gall bladder disease, thromboembolic disease, estrogen dependent tumors of the breast, and endometrial carcinoma. He described very few significant adverse effects in his patients ("20 years experience and . . . more than 700 published cases"). He also noted, it seems somewhat defensively, that "most patients complaining of side effects are neurotic or are placebo reactors" (p. 3).

Adverse effects and therapeutic limitations would appear to constitute significant issues in the use of estrogen therapy. The positive gains in relief of vasomotor symptoms, atrophic vaginitis, and some psychological distress are impressive. However, the extent to which estrogens can improve depression remains controversial. In light of the overall findings, short-term low-dose use in patients for whom vasomotor symptoms are present would seem most advisable. Total dose received and length of treatment require particular attention in subsequent research. The relative cost, risk, and benefit may be found to change substantially as a function of the length of the course of estrogen treatment.

## CONCLUSIONS AND RECOMMENDATIONS

The appreciation that menopausal distress is a psychosomatic phenomenon is perhaps the strongest conclusion from current research. Viewing psychosomatic phenomena as those in which both physical and psychological factors contribute to the genesis, maintenance, and treatment (Selby & Calhoun, 1978; Wright, 1977), both menstrual and menopausal symptoms emerge as common examples. Although it is important for research efforts to attempt to disentangle the contributions of biological factors and psychological factors, it is apparent that clinicians need to be sensitive to the interrelatedness of both sets of factors in treating individual patients.

Sensitivity to emotional symptoms, interpersonal worries, and sexual concerns of climacteric patients seems especially warranted. The quite notable improvement with placebo observed in many estrogen treatment studies reinforces the importance of emotional support and reassurance in treatment. Placebo response, with relief of symptomatic distress, does not imply that the symptom relieved was psychogenetic. For example, postoperative surgical pain, and pain associated with a variety of other physical conditions, can often be effectively relieved by placebo. Placebo responders, constituting about one third of most populations studied, are neither more neurotic nor less intelligent than general populations. Indeed, preliminary research (Levine, Gordon & Fields, 1978) has suggested that placebo may act, at least with respect to pain, through endorphin (naturally occurring opiate-like substances in the brain) mediated pathways.

In the clinical treatment of menopausal women, along with whatever physical measures seem advisable, psychosocial elements must be emphasized. The treatment of menopausal patients is a prime area for the collaboration of general physicians and obstetricians with psychiatrists, psychologists, counselors, and social workers in both clinical practice and research endeavors.

In working with women experiencing menopausal difficulties, a psychodidactic approach with emphasis on conveying personally relevant information (Selby & Calhoun, in press) would seem desirable. Information concerning the common psychological, social, and physical changes associated with the climacteric period might help the distressed woman gain a better understanding of her situation, reduce the impact of negative social attitudes and expectations, and reduce uncertainty and misconceptions on her part. The conveying of such information can be easily incorporated into most treatment regimes and seems likely to help mitigate discomfort.

As population trends shift toward a greater proportion of older individuals, attitudes and beliefs about the menopause assume greater social importance. What once marked the onset of old age has now become an event of midlife. However, as the sex role expectations of women broaden, and they gain greater freedom from reproductive functions, the relative significance of the menopause is likely to diminish. As Osofsky and Seidenberg (1970) observed, "Sexuality, reproduction and childbearing may be important to both males and females but should be choices and not mandated at the exclusion of other avenues of fulfillment for women" (p. 614).

## REFERENCES

Adamopoulis, D. A., Loraine, J. A., and Dove, G. A. Endocrinological studies in women approaching the menopause. *Journal of Obstetrics and Gynecology of the British Commonwealth,* 1971, *78,* 62–79.

Aitken, J. M. Osteoporosis and its relation to estrogen deficiency. In S. Campbell (ed.), *The management of the menopause and post-menopausal years.* Baltimore: University Park Press, 1976.

Albright, F., and Reinfenstein, E. C. *The parathyroid glands in metabolic bone disease.* Baltimore: The Williams & Wilkins Co., 1949.

Andor, J. Possibilites du traitement hormonal des troubles climateriques definies en considerant plus particulierement une nouvelle methode de administration orale des oestrogenes. *Revue Therapeutique* 31:182, 1974.

Antunes, C. M., Stolley, P. D., Rosenshein, N. B., Davis, J. L. Tonascia, J. A., Brown, C., Burnett, L., Rutledge, A., Pokempner, M., and Garcia, R., Endometrial cancer and estrogen use. *New England Journal of Medicine,* 1979, *300,* 9–13.

Aylward, M. Estrogen, plasma tryptophan in perimenopausal patients. In S. Campbell (ed.), *The management of the menopause and post-menopausal years.* Baltimore: University Park Press, 1976.

Ballinger, C. B. Psychiatric aspects of the menopause. In S. Campbell (ed.), *The management of the menopause and post-menopause years.* Baltimore: University Park Press, 1976.

———. Psychiatric morbidity and the menopause: clinical features. *British Medical Journal,* 1976, 1(6019), 1183–1185.

———. Psychiatric morbidity and the menopause: screening of a general population sample. *British Medical Journal,* 1975, 3(5979), 344–346.

———. Psychiatric morbidity and the menopause: survey of a gynecological outpatient clinic. *British Journal of Psychiatry,* 1977, *131,* 83–89.

BLOOD, R. O., and WOLFE, D. M. *Husbands and wives: the dynamics of married living.* New York: Free Press, 1960.

BOSSARD, J. H. S., and BOLL, E. S. Marital unhappiness in the life cycle of marriage. *Marriage and Family Living,* 1955, *17,* 10.

BRANSOME, E. D. Medical complications of estrogens and oral contraceptives. In R. B. Greenblatt (ed.), *The menopausal syndrome.* New York: Medicom, 1974.

BROWN, M. D. Emotional response to the menopause. In S. Campbell (ed.), *The management of the menopause and post-menopausal years.* Baltimore: University Park Press, 1976.

BURR, W. R. Satisfaction with marriage over the life cycle. *Journal of Marriage and the Family,* 1970, *32,* 29.

CALHOUN, L. G., SELBY, J. W., and KING, E. *Dealing with crisis.* Englewood Cliffs: Prentice-Hall, 1976.

CAMPBELL, S. (ed.). *The management of the menopause and post-menopausal years.* Baltimore: University Park Press, 1976.

CAMPBELL, S., and WHITEHEAD, M. Oestrogen therapy and the menopausal syndrome. *Clinical Obstetrics and Gynaecology,* 1977, *4,* 31–47.

COOPE, J. Double blind cross-over study of estrogen replacement therapy. In S. Campbell (ed.), *The management of the menopause and post-menopausal years.* Baltimore: University Park Press, 1976.

COOPER, W. Hormone replacement therapy. *Royal Society of Health Journal,* 1976, *96,* 81–85.

COPE, E. Physical changes associated with the post-menopausal years. In S. Campbell (ed.), *The management of the menopause & postmenopausal years.* Baltimore: University Park Press, 1976.

DAPUNT, O. Behandlung klimakterischer beschwerden mit ostradiolvalirianat. (Progynova) Medizinische Klinik 62:1356–1361, 1967.

DEUTSCH, H. *The psychology of women.* New York: Grune & Stratton, 1945.

DEUTSCHER, I. *Married life in the middle years.* Kansas City: Missouri Community Studies, 1959.

DEWHURST, C. J. Frequency and severity of menopausal symptoms. In S. Campbell (ed.), *The management of the menopause and post-menopausal years.* Baltimore: University Park Press, 1976.

DEYKIN, E. Y. The empty nest psychosocial aspects of conflict between depressed women and their grown children. *American Journal of Psychiatry,* 1966, *122,* 1422.

DOMINIAN, J. The role of psychiatry in the menopause. *Clinics in Obstetrics and Gynecology,* 1977, *4,* 241–257.

FEDOR-FREYBERGH, P. The influence of oestrogens on the wellbeing and mental performance in climacteric and post-menopausal women. *Acta Obstetricia et Gynecologica Scandanavica,* 1977, *64,* 1–91.

FLINT, M. Cross-cultural factors that affect age of menopause. In *Consensus on menopause research.* Baltimore: University Park Press, 1976.

FREUD, S. Mourning and melancholia. In John D. Sutherland (ed.), *Collected Papers* (vol. 4). London: The Hogarth Press and the Institute of Psycho-Analysis, 1925.

GALLOWAY, K. The change of life. *American Journal of Nursing,* 1975, *75,* 1006–1011.

GREENBLATT, R. B., MAHESH, V. B., and MCDONOUGH, P. G. *The menopausal syndrome.* New York: Medicom, 1974.

HAUSER, G. A., DAHINDEN, U., SAMARTZIS, S., and WENNER, R. Effects and side-effects of oestrogen therapy on the climacture syndrome. In P. A. Van Keep and C. Lauritzen (eds.), *Ageing and estrogens.* Frontiers of Hormone Research, vol. 2. Basel: Karger, 1973.

HAUSER, G. A., and WENNER, R. Die endokrine umstelling im klimakterium. *Therapeutische Umschau,* 1974, *31,* 155.

HENKER, F. O. Sexual, psychic, and physical complaints in 50 middle-aged men. *Psychosomatics,* 1977, *18,* 23–27.

HUMPHREY, M. The empty nest syndrome: theoretical considerations. Paper presented to the International Congress on the Menopause, La Grande Motte, 1976.

JASZMANN, L. J. B. Epidemiology of the climacteric syndrome. In S. Campbell (ed.), *The management of the menopause and post-menopausal years.* Baltimore: University Park Press, 1976.

JASZMANN, L. J. B., VAN LITH, W. D., and ZAAL, J. C. A. The age of menopause in the Netherlands. *International Journal of Fertility,* 1969, *14,* 106.

JEFFCOATE, T. N. A. Drugs for menopausal symptoms. *British Medical Journal,* 1960, no. 5169, 340–342.

JICK, H., WATKINS, R. N., HUNTER, J. R., DINAN, B., MADSEN, S., ROTHMAN, K., and WALKER, A. Replacement estrogens and endometrial cancer. *New England Journal of Medicine,* 1979, *300,* 218–222.

KIELHOLZ, P. Diagnosis and therapy of the depressive states. *Documentum Geigy Acta Psychosomatica* (North America), 1959, no. 1, 37. In A. M. Freedman, H. I. Kaplan, and B. J. Sadock (eds.), *Comprehensive textbook of psychiatry,* Vol. 2 (2nd ed.). Baltimore: Williams & Wilkins Co., 1975.

KERR, M. D. Psychohormonal approach to the menopause. *Modern Treatment,* 1968, *5,* 587.

———. Psychological changes following hormonal therapy. In S. Campbell (ed.), *The management of the menopause and post-menopausal years.* Baltimore: University Park Press, 1976.

KINSEY, A. C., POMEROY, W. B., and MORTON, C. E. *Sexual behavior in the human male.* Philadelphia: Saunders, 1948.

KLAIBER, E. L., BROVERMAN, D. M., VOGEL, W., and KOBAYASHI, Y. The use of steroid hormones in depression. In T. M. Itel, G. Laundahn, and W. Hermann (eds.), *Psychotropic action of hormones.* New York: Spectrum, 1976.

KLAIBER, E. L., KOBAYASHI, Y., BROVERMAN, D. M., and HALL, T. Plasma monoamine oxidase activity in regularly menstruating women and in amenorrheic women receiving cyclic treatment with estrogens and a progestin. *Journal of Clinical Endocrinology and Metabolism,* 1971, *33,* 630.

LANG, N. Pathogenese, diagnostic und behandlung klimakterischer beschwerden. *Gynakologe,* 1970, *2,* 122.

LAURITZEN, C. The female climacteric with special reference to disturbances of the diencephalopituitary control mechanism. *Journal of Neurovisceral Relations,* 1971, (supplement 10) (644).

———. The hypothalamic anterior pituitary system in the climacteric age period. In P. A. Van Keep and C. Lauritzen (eds.), *Estrogens in the post-menopause.* Frontiers of Hormone Research, vol. 3. Basel: Karger, 1975.

———. The estrogen deficiency syndrome and the management of the patient. In S. Campbell (ed.), *The management of the menopause and post-menopausal years.* Baltimore: University Park Press, 1976.

LEBECH, P. E. Hormone therapy of the menopause: a panel. In Greenblatt, R. B., Mahesh, V. B., and McDonough, P. G. (eds.), *The menopausal syndrome.* New York: Medicom, 1974.

LEVINE, J. D., GORDON, N. C., and FIELDS, H. L. The mechanism of placebo analgesia. *Lancet,* 1978, *2,* 654–657.

LIDZ, T. The family as the developmental setting. In C. J. Anthony and C. Koupernik (eds.), *The child in his family.* New York: Wiley, 1970.

LOZMAN, H., BARLOW, M. D., and LEVITT, D. G. Piperazine estrone sulfate and conjugated estrogens equine in the treatment of the menopausal syndrome. *Southern Medical Journal,* 1971, *64,* 1143–1149.

MACK, T., PIKE, M., HENDERSON, B., PFEFFER, R., GERKINS, V., ARTHUR, M., and BROWN, S. Estrogens and endometrial cancer in a retirement community. *New England Journal of Medicine,* 1976, *294,* 1262.

MCCANDLESS, F. D. Emotional problems of the climacteric. *Clinical Obstetrics and Gynecology,* 1964, *17,* 489.

MCEWAN, J. A. Menopause: myths and medicine. *Nursing Times,* 1973, *69,* 1483–1484.

MCKINLAY, S. M., and JEFFERYS, M. The menopausal syndrome. *British Journal of Preventative Social Medicine,* 1974, *28,* 108–115.

MCKINLAY, S. M., and MCKINLAY, J. K. Selected studies of the menopause. *Journal of Biosocial Science,* 1973, *5,* 589.

NEUGARTEN, B. L., and KRAINES, R. J. Menopausal symptoms in women of various ages. *Psychosomatic Medicine,* 1965, *28,* 266–273.

NIKULA-BAUMANN, L. Endocrinological studies on subjects with involutional melancholia. *Acta Psychiatrica Scandanavica,* 1971, *226,* 107.

OSBORNE, N. L. Post-menopausal changes in menstruation habits and in urine flow and urethral pressure studies. In *MM and PM years.* Baltimore: University Park Press, 1976.

OSOFSKY, H. J., and SEIDENBERG, R. Is female menopausal depression inevitable? *Obstetrics and Gynecology,* 1970, *36,* 611–615.

PINEO, P. C. Disenchantment in the later years of marriage. *Journal of Marriage and the Family,* 1961, *23,* 3.

PRATT, J. P., and THOMAS, W. L. The endocrine treatment of menopausal phenomena. *Journal of the American Medical Association,* 1937, *109,* 1875.

RADMAYR, E. Die steroidhormone in klimakterium. *Wiener Medizinische Wochenschrift,* 1970, *48,* 903.

ROLLINS, B. C., and FELDMAN, H. Marital satisfaction over the family life cycle. *Journal of Marriage and the Family,* 1970, *32,* 20.

SCHNEIDER, M. A., BROTHERTON, P. L., and HAILES, J. The effect of exogenous estrogens on depression in menopausal women. *Medical Journal of Australia,* 1977, *2,* 162–163.

SEGALOFF, A. The metabolism of estrogens with particular emphasis on clinical aspects of physiology and function of ovarian hormones. *Recent Progress in Hormone Research,* 1949, *4,* 85.

SELBY, J. W., and CALHOUN, L. G. Psychosomatic phenomena: an extension of Wright. *American Psychologist,* 1978, *33,* 396–398.

SELBY, J. W. and CALHOUN, L. G. The psychodidactic element of psychological intervention: an undervalued and underdeveloped treatment tool. *Professional Psychology,* 1980, *11,* 236–241.

SMITH, D. C., PRENTICE, R., THOMPSON, D., and HERMANN, W. Association of exogenous estrogen and endometrial carcinoma. *New England Journal of Medicine,* 1975, *293,* 1164.

Smith, P. J. B. The effect of estrogens on bladder function in the female. In *The management of the menopause and post-menopausal years.* Baltimore: University Park Press, 1976.

Spicer, C. C., Hare, S. A., and Slater, E. Neurotic and psychotic forms of depressive illness. *British Journal of Psychiatry,* 1973, *123,* 53.

Thompson, B., Hart, S. A., and Durno, D. Menopausal age and symptomatology in a general practise. *Journal of Biosocial Sciences,* 1973, *5,* 71.

Thompson, J. Double blind study on the effect of estrogen on sleep, anxiety, and depression in perimenopausal women: preliminary results. *Proceedings of the Royal Society of Medicine,* 1976, *69,* 829–830.

Utian, W. H. Current status of menopause and postmenopausal estrogen therapy. *Obstetrics and Gynecology Survey,* 1977, *32,* 193–204.

Van Keep, P. A., and Humphrey, M. Psycho-social aspects of the climacteric. In P. A. Van Keep (eds.), *Consensus on menopause research.* Baltimore: University Park Press, 1976.

Wilson, R. A., and Wilson, T. A. The fate of the nontreated post menopausal woman: a plea for the maintenance of adequate estrogen from puberty to the grave. *Journal of American Geriatrics,* 1963, *11,* 347.

Winokur, G. Depression in the menopause. *American Journal of Psychiatry,* 1973, *130,* 92–93.

Winter, G. F. Naturliche konjugierte ostrogene in klimakterium. *Zentralbl Gynaekal,* 1967, *89,* 296–300.

Wright, L. Conceptualizing and defining psychosomatic disorders. *American Psychologist,* 1977, *32,* 625–628.

Ziel, H., and Finkle, W. Increased risk of endometrial carcinoma among users of conjugated estrogen. *New England Journal of Medicine,* 1975, *293,* 1167.

# Index

9 781416 577713